INTERMITTENT FASTING

Table of Contents

INTRODUCTION

Intermittent fasting (IF) is an eating method that allows people to restrict their food intake for 16–24 hours. Intermittent fasting can help burn fat and lose weight. It would be best if you only did intermittent fasting when you have a well-planned, healthy eating plan in place. However, it is not for everyone, so it's essential to understand the short- and long-term benefits before you embark on the program.

The term intermittent fasting is a bit of a misnomer. Intermittent fasting doesn't mean that you're going without food for one day every week or one month every year. Instead, it's a more descriptive term for a nutrition pattern you regularly eat for brief periods. The science behind intermittent fasting has been explored by some of the world's leading researchers in recent years, and there are now many health benefits to be found. Simply put, intermittent fasting is eating during shorter periods of your day—between 4–12 hours—with no specific eating window. Instead of eating throughout the day as most people do, you'll break your usual eating window into three or four shorter "snacks" throughout the day. It will allow you to get more nutritional value out of each meal, plus it will be harder to overeat or mindlessly snack between meals. A fast is a short-term limitation of calories typically followed by a period of normal eating—intermittent fasting. It's a way to improve health and reduce the likelihood of chronic diseases potentially.

Intermittent fasting can help you feel fuller sooner because it tricks your body into thinking that it's not getting food when you're fasting. The type of intermittent fasting you choose depends on what works best for your body's unique needs. Your doctor can help you find the most suitable, irregular fasting plan for your lifestyle, goals, and medical conditions. Intermittent fasting can be a practical dieting strategy if you are trying to lose weight or improve your health. However, not everyone can do it, as it takes willpower and discipline to avoid eating when tempted by other foods.

Fasting has been a treatment for various medical conditions, including diabetes, obesity, heart disease, and high cholesterol. Most people in the western world have never heard of fasting before, so intermittent fasting is appealing. It was maybe as simple as eating only for a few hours each day, or sometimes taking several days off from eating altogether. That's right, no food for three or five days at a time! With intermittent fasting, you don't need to feel restricted by your daily caloric intake. Get started on your new lifestyle today!

CHAPTER 1: INTERMITTENT FASTING AND WHY IT IS GOOD FOR YOU

Intermittent fasting is fasting when you keep away any kind of foodstuff involving calories among ordinary nutritious ingredients. It is not starvation or a way for you to eat junk food with no consequences. There are various methods used to practice IF; they divide time into hours or divide time into days. Since the response to the regiment varies from person to person, no process can be called the best.

Intermittent fasting cannot make you lose those additional pounds instantaneously, but it can prevent unhealthy addictions. It's a nutritional practice that requires you to be determined to follow it and get the desired result. If you already have little time for eating due to your schedule, this regiment will suit you like a duck to water, but you will always need to be conscious of what you are eating. Choose the appropriate regiment after you take expert guidance. You should see it as a segment of your schedule to get healthy, but not the only component.

If you do it frequently, your body becomes used to it; thus, it automatically becomes a regular practice for you. Your body will alter your hunger patterns, as you'll feel famished when you're ready to eat rather than following false hunger signals. When intermittent fasting is done for more extended periods, it ends in quicker results, but long fasts are done less frequently. It is possible to switch plans, but don't do it because you find it hard initially, as all of them are quite similar.

You're eating patterns influence hormones that increase appetite and fat retention, like insulin. The quantity of food and the eating time affect your circadian rhythms. These circadian rhythms are predictable recurrent variations of hormone levels over a day—nearly all hormones, like those required for growth.

The circadian rhythms are affected by the season and time of the day. Food was most likely available during the day in the Paleolithic period, as they used the sunlight for hunting because they had no light source at night. Other animals have inverted circadian rhythms because they hunt at night and sleep in the day. You may consume the same meals, but the timing can create a considerable variation in your body and general wellness. In the evening, the insulin levels are higher than in the morning, so eating large meals can cause more fat to be stored in your body. It helps connect the relationship between eating and obesity since it is more of a hormonal inequality than calorific inequality.

If you are in a heavily stressed environment, intermittent fasting can be challenging. It can do the opposite of what you want it to do as it can increase fat storage.

Believe it or not, a circadian rhythm was followed by hunger; otherwise, we would be hungry all the time. Need is lowest in the morning, and desire is at its highest at night. Hormones affect when you feel hungry, so the period you have stayed without eating doesn't matter. It takes time for hormones to adjust so that you may feel hungry during the first few days of fasting, but after that, you will not feel hungry during your time of fasting.

Many people say that breakfast is supposed to be the largest meal of the day, but in fact, you're the least hungry in the morning, as stated earlier. Eating a large breakfast is just forcing the body to eat food that it doesn't need; it hurts your weight loss goals. Your insulin concentrations are highest at night, leading to a lot of glucose converting into fat; thus, more fat is stored when you eat a large meal in the evening. Lunchtime is the optimum time to eat the largest meal of the day.

During a diet, burning up stored fats is the way the body gets energy. It will teach your body to use fats for strength and forfeit glucose, even when you're not fasting. In organs like the heart and lungs, your body utilizes stored fat for energy, but more is generated due to unnecessary eating. Also, organs using recycled fat do not have enough time to use that fat as glucose is carried continuously into the system, so the body first needs to get rid of it. If you eat a lot and do not exercise, your body cells cannot burn the stored fat.

By default, the cells of a healthy person are designed to burn fat for energy, so intermittent fasting is like adding gasoline to a fire. Encouraging your system to make fat—your only energy source—will help you lose more fat in the long run. Exercise can help you with this process. Training allows your cells to consume fat and glucose when the body needs it, providing you energy rather than enhancing fat retention.

History of Fasting

According to the American Heart Association, intermittent fasting may be an effective way to lose weight, increase your metabolism, and increase longevity. This method involves periods of fasting that can range from 16 hours to 24 hours every day.

Although intermittent fasting is a new idea to most people, it certainly isn't a new concept. The most widely known version of it is called the "5:2 diet." In this diet, you eat 500 calories for some time, restricting your calorie intake to 600 calories for 2 days and then allowing yourself to eat up to 1,000 calories a day for the remaining 5 days.

Historically, humans have been doing intermittent fasting ever since they began eating food. There are many different kinds of fasting that have been practiced since ancient times. In some cases, minimal amounts of food or water were intermittently withheld from the body. For instance, when a person was in distress, fasting could provide spiritual and physical benefits. Many cultures still practice fasting worldwide today, such as in the Muslim world where laws require Muslims to fast at least once per year during Ramadan.

Advantage of Intermittent Fasting

There are a lot of advantages to intermittent fasting. First and foremost, it is a weight-loss method that allows you to eat whatever you want—within reason—while maintaining a healthy diet. You don't have to follow a strict exercise routine or count calories to lose weight. There are other benefits as well, such as increased energy, better mental clarity, and more! All you have to do is to learn how to do it properly.

It means that you don't have to skip meals to lose weight. You can eat all the food you want without any harm to your metabolism or health. Intermittent fasting is not difficult to learn if you follow the guide that we've provided.

Who Should Not Fast?

Some people should not fast. If you have a medical condition or are pregnant, please speak with a physician before starting a fast. Understand that fasting can cause more harm than good. Many people engage in intermittent fasting to control their weight, and so you could experience adverse side effects if you're not aware of them.

The Myth of Fasting

Fasting sounds like a great idea, but it's a myth that could be dangerous to your health. Fasting for extended periods is linked to a higher risk of death and many health conditions.

Health Benefits from Intermittent Fasting

People are drawn to the idea of intermittent fasting because it can help with weight loss. The advantage of this method is that you typically don't feel hungry, which means you are more likely to stick to your diet.

However, you don't have to go with the whole 24-hour fast to get these benefits. A shorter 20-hour fast or a 16-hour fast are safe alternatives that could be effective at helping you lose weight. All you need is 5 days of fasting for over 4 weeks.

But intermittent fasting isn't just about dropping pounds; it's also used to treat many other health conditions. Some examples include:

Insulin Resistance: One study found that fasting for people who have insulin resistance can decrease insulin levels in the blood, improving their insulin sensitivity.

High Cholesterol: Intermittent fasting has been shown in studies to improve high cholesterol levels without any adverse effects on HDL (good cholesterol) levels. The study showed a decrease in total cholesterol and LDL (bad) cholesterol following an 8-week fast. Another study found four weeks of intermittent fasting increased HDL levels (good cholesterol) and decreased LDL levels.

Fasting for Diabetes

There are essential health benefits to intermittent fasting.

You may not be aware, but intermittent fasting has been used for centuries to reduce the risk of developing type II diabetes and other diseases.

You can do intermittent fasting by merely skipping meals. Studies have shown that this may play an essential role in reducing your heart disease risk, diabetes, cancer, and many other chronic diseases.

Some people like to fast by eating only from 9 a.m. and 3 p.m. Others prefer to fast for 16 hours, or from 6 p.m. until 11 p.m. The main thing is to try some different intermittent fasting schedules and see what works best for you.

Fasting for Heart Health

Fasting may be the only way to get all the ketogenic diet benefits without dietary restrictions. Intermittent fasting can help improve heart health, shed weight, and increase energy levels.

Here's why: Intermittent fasting can help improve heart health because it increases your body's fat-burning potential by forcing the body to burn stored fat rather than glucose.

If your goal is to lose weight, intermittent fasting can lead to fewer calories consumed each day, potentially decreasing hunger and giving you more energy and focus throughout the day. It can also slash blood sugar levels, making it easier for you to maintain healthy blood sugar levels with less insulin resistance and a healthier metabolism.

CHAPTER 2: HOW TO FAST

Fasting is a natural way of regulating your body's metabolism. It can benefit your health, and it can help you achieve your weight loss goals. Conventional wisdom has it that if you want to lose weight, it's best to fast for a couple of days and normally eat for the remainder of the week.

In reality, intermittent fasting is more effective than long-term calorie restriction. Here's how it works:

If you eat less than 500 calories per day, you're not going to lose much weight at all. You might not lose any! That's because your body takes a while to respond to a calorie shortage. During this time, you become less active, which causes your metabolism to slow down.

Intermittent fasting allows your body to avoid this problem by restricting calories for a short period (usually 6–12 hours) and then allowing yourself to eat normally again for the remainder of the day. By following this routine, you can potentially enjoy the benefits of intermittent fasting while still maintaining a healthy diet and losing weight at a reasonable rate.

Here are some recommendations for how to go about intermittent fasting:

Fast Every Other Day: On non-fasting days, try eating only 500 calories per day or less. If you prefer a higher caloric intake, start with 600 calories per day and work your way down from there as needed. If possible, try fasting on consecutive days by eating 500 calories on a fast day and then consuming an unlimited food allowance for the remainder of the week.

Fast One Day: Follow the same method as above, but only fast on 1 day per week instead of two.

Alternate Days: Instead of alternating between fast days and nonfasting days, try cycling between 2 different types of fasting cycles to maximize fat loss while minimizing muscle loss.

Kinds of Fasting

Intermittent fasting is a fasting method in which you usually eat only during the times between your regular eating times. Here are two types of intermittent fasting:

- Alternate-day fasting (ADF)
- Alternate-day alternating fasting (ADAF)

Don't let the terms confuse you. The key is to pick an intermittent fasting routine that works best for your lifestyle. It's also essential to find one that doesn't make you feel deprived or guilty during regular eating times.

Dieters do an ADF by skipping breakfast and only eating during their regular eating times. If you usually eat breakfast at 8 a.m., then miss it and only eat again at 9 a.m., and that would be an ADF routine for you. Always take a look at your schedule and choose a meal schedule that works best for you before diving into your intermittent fasting routine.

If skipping breakfast sounds like too big of a change to make, try out AADA instead. With AADA, you only eat during your standard eating times and then fast for 12–36 hours every other day or every third day. You start your eating window on the first day of a new month, so start it on 1/1/2013 and end it on 1/14/2013 (for example). On the other days of the month, skip breakfast and immediately eat again after 8 p.m. or resume your regular eating schedule. You're eating window will go from 1/1/2013 to 1/14/2013 (for example). Experiment with different eating windows to find what works best for you!

Intermittent Fasting Best Practices

Intermittent fasting is a technique that involves limiting the amount of food you eat during some days of your week. This practice mimics the starvation periods of our ancestors.

The idea behind intermittent fasting is that the body becomes more efficient at extracting energy from food. This diet works for many people, but there are some best practices that you'll want to follow if you decide to tinker with this diet.

Recent research has shown that you start to react to how much food you need to change your eating habits. Most people tend to eat more in the afternoon and at night, whereas they feel hungry first thing in the morning. It is because our body processes food differently throughout the day and through each meal.

By limiting your intake slightly throughout the day, your body will get better at maintaining energy levels between meals. It means that you'll have a better chance of not feeling hungry when it's time for lunch or dinner.

Water Fasting and Different Types of Fasting

You're probably wondering how intermittent fasting works. Intermittent fasting is a simple eating pattern that you can use to achieve optimal health and lose weight. In a nutshell, it means you eat in a certain way on specified days and don't eat at all on others.

The first type of intermittent fasting is known as water fasting. Here, you consume only water at least once every 24 hours. You must continue to consume fluids such as black tea or coffee. This method of fasting helps your body release stored fat while simultaneously keeping you satisfied and energized.

The second type of fasting is intermittent fasting. This type includes alternate day fasting, time-restricted eating, and meal skipping. With alternate day fasting, you eat for 5 consecutive days each week. During the other 2 days of the week, you fast. Time-restricted eating limits the amount of food you eat and the time you spend eating. Meal skipping dictates that you only eat 3 meals each day. If you choose to eat quickly during these 3 meals (breakfast, lunch, and dinner), you will burn calories during the day and have a better chance of losing weight than if you ate all 5 meals throughout the day.

Longer and Extended Periods of Fasting

Most people may know a little about intermittent fasting, but not a lot. "What is intermittent fasting and how long should I fast?" is one of the most common questions we hear. Intermittent fasting is, essentially, going without food for a certain period, like 16 hours for your fasting period and 8 hours for your eating window.

Most intermittent fasts last between 12–24 hours. It can range from 4–24 hours, depending on the individual. Generally, sporadic fasts are much less restrictive than typical 16-hour fasts, as they may only last 12 hours. It isn't to say that they're comfortable because you have to make sure you stay hydrated and complete your exercises during this period.

Extended fasting is the same as intermittent fasting, except that you don't fast for extended periods. You limit your caloric intake to a small amount at certain times during the day and then go back to the regular eating pattern when the fasting period is over.

Since food can't enter your body without calories, the only way to get rid of fat is to burn energy reserves accumulated from the calories you consume. It will help you burn away those unwanted pounds while getting healthy at the same time. It's a win-win!

Fasting Tips

Fasting is a controversial topic. Some people believe that it can cure cancer; others think that it's a waste of time.

For those of you who need to lose weight, you should know some essential things. Here are the top tips with intermittent fasting:

Eat on an Empty Stomach: Fasting makes your body go into "starvation mode," so if you eat on an empty stomach, you'll be better able to digest your meals and get the most out of them.

Aim for a 25–40% Daily Caloric Intake Fast: It will depend on how much weight you want to lose.

Eat When You're Hungry and Stop When You're Full: Don't force yourself to eat if you aren't hungry, and don't starve yourself if you're full by overeating. Your body will work as best as it can when you fast, so trust your instincts. If your stomach feels full, stop eating, move on with your day, or have a snack if you still feel hungry.

Keep Your Blood Sugar at Normal Levels: By drinking water and doing things like chewing gum or drinking vitamin water, you will prevent your body from breaking down muscle for energy during the fast, and you'll gain weight during the immediate rather than lose weight.

Coffee Isn't Good for Fasting: It's quick energy that keeps your blood sugar level up, and if you're trying to lose weight or are fasting for medical reasons, it can lead to cravings and hunger pangs, which will kick-start the "starvation mode" scenario described above.

Watch out for Dinner: It is often the most challenging meal of the day due to hunger pangs and cravings. The trick is not to overeat here; try not to devour more than 1 large portion for each meal.

CHAPTER 3: FASTING PROTOCOL

There are many varieties of intermittent fasting. Some involve eating every other day or eating once every 3 days.

Most of the intermittent fasting protocols I've seen focus on skipping breakfast. Still, other variations exist, such as eating only once a day or limiting your daily caloric intake to 500–800 calories.

One of the popular intermittent fasting protocols is the one that focuses on eating every 16 hours. It can be done daily and on special days where you might want to go longer than 16 hours without eating. It's best to leave at least 12 hours between regularly scheduled meals to keep your metabolism high and to allow your body to rest from digesting food—all of its associated metabolic byproducts.

Protocols

We are continually changing as we grow, grow old, and get sick. The downside of these changes is that it's difficult to know how much fat you should have. How much fat you should have can vary from person to person, so it's hard to know what your daily calorie intake should be. It can lead to strategies like crash diets, where you're losing weight quickly and getting no benefit from the effort. Crash diets and other methods may even lead to nutrient deficiencies, making you more susceptible to infections and other health risks.

Intermittent fasting protocols allow you to lose weight healthily by controlling your daily calorie intake without restricting calories below your body's needs. We recommend intermittent fasting protocols for both men and women looking for a healthy way to weight loss.

Many people are interested in an intermittent fasting diet. The protocol is as follows:

Do not eat for 16 hours from the time of your last meal. It is known as your fasting window. You can consume water or other beverages during this period, but make sure they are different from any foods you have finished. You can also have snacks at any time during your fast, but these should be no more than 500 calories.

After your first 16-hour fast, there is no strict boundary on when you may start eating again. However, it is said that after about 24 hours of eating, you will begin to get hungry and will begin to break the fast. It means you should start eating after you think you are no longer hungry and stop eating before you are so hungry that you cannot function. It's essential to do this because if it causes you to miss days of work or school, it could become a problem.

The benefits of intermittent fasting include rapid weight loss management, hormonal balance, and improved physical performance. Almost everyone knows that fasting reduces levels of the hunger hormone ghrelin, which helps with weight loss. Another benefit is that while intermittent fasting causes the body to burn fat as fuel, it also lowers insulin sensitivity, which will help stabilize blood sugar levels. Most people find that after doing an extended fast several times, they become much less sensitive to insulin and require lower doses of insulin and medications such as metformin to control diabetes. This strategy also leads to weight loss.

Start by figuring out your ideal fasting time. Ideally, it would help if you were consuming within an 8-hour window around the time you plan to fast. It can be achieved by setting your alarm clock to a time that will allow you to begin fasting when you wake up in the morning and end 8 hours later.

Once you have your ideal fasting window figured out, create a way to avoid consuming any food or drink within that window. If this is not possible, then there are several options available to help you break the fast:

Beverages: A fast can be broken if someone is consuming water or other nonexotic beverage within the first 8 hours after waking. These drinks should not contain more than 0.4 oz. of fat per 16 oz. (in a bottle) since fat content will affect the number of calories absorbed in the 24 hours and slightly increase this period length. You may drink coffee/tea or other nonalcoholic beverages during this period to help yourself burn fat and speed up recovery. Remember, do not consume any additional calories or nutrients during this period, as they will reset your 24-hours fast to the beginning of the day.

Water/Nutrient: A fast can be broken if someone is consuming 800 mg of water a day, or another nonexotic nutrient within the first 8 hours after waking. These drinks should contain no more than 20% fat content, and 1,000 mg of sodium per 16 oz. (in a bottle) since fat content will affect the number of calories absorbed in 24 hours and slightly increase this period length. Once again, coffee/tea or other nonalcoholic beverages (that do not contain alcohol) can fill in small gaps without much harm if you decide to go with it.

A common question we get to ask is about the intermittent fasting protocols, so we've compiled a few different fasting protocols for your convenience.

Intermittent fasting protocols are essential to follow, as they can produce tremendous health benefits. Many studies have shown that intermittent fasting can help protect your body from disease and promote improved health.

The benefits of intermittent fasting are numerous, and they start with weight loss. Intermittent fasting helps in melting fat cells without losing muscle tissue, and it boosts your metabolic rate, which in turn reduces your appetite. Intermittent fasting also speeds up your metabolism, improving your overall health and making you look younger. That means fewer calories for you to eat—and fewer calories for you to store as fat.

While intermittent fasting does not cause weight loss on its own, it is an excellent tool for weight loss, and it can help you keep off the weight you do lose. It's no wonder why our customers love intermittent fasting!

CHAPTER 4: INTERMITTENT FASTING POTENTIAL DOWNSIDES

Anxiety Attacks

Another potential side effect of detoxing through intermittent fasting is the potential for an anxiety attack. It can happen when you are withholding food for an extended period, especially if you are new to intermittent fasting.

An anxiety attack may come upon you because you feel that you are not getting enough nutrition or missing your usual feeding times.

Digestive Distress

Since intermittent fasting has a detoxing component, you may experience digestive distress during your first few experiences. It is due to your body flushing out much of the residual matter in your body in addition to merely excreting whatever is still leftover in the digestive tract.

As long as it isn't anything that you feel abnormal, you can attribute it to the detoxing process. However, if symptoms do not subside, then you may need to seek medical attention at once.

You Might Struggle to Maintain Blood Sugar Levels

Although the intermittent fasting diet tends to improve blood sugar levels in most people, this is not always true for everyone. Some people following the intermittent fasting diet may find that their ability to maintain a healthy blood sugar level is compromised.

The reason why this happens varies. For some people, not eating frequently enough may encourage this to happen. For others, transitioning too quickly or taking on too intense of a fasting cycle too soon can result in a shock to the body that causes a strange fluctuation in blood sugar levels.

You Might Experience Hormonal Imbalances

A certain degree of fasting, especially when you build up to it, can support you in having healthier hormone levels. However, for some people, intermittent fasting may lead to an unhealthy imbalance of hormones. It can result in many different hormone-based symptoms, such as headaches, fatigue, and even menstrual problems in women.

Again, the reason for the hormonal imbalance varies. For some people, particularly those who are already at risk of experiencing hormonal imbalances, intermittent fasting can trigger these imbalances. For others, it could go back to what they are consuming during the eating windows. Eating meals that are not rich in nutrients and vitamins can result in you not having enough nutrition to support your hormonal levels.

If you begin experiencing hormonal imbalances while you follow the intermittent fasting diet, you must stop and consult your doctor right away. Discovering where the shortcomings are and how you can correct them is vital. Having imbalanced hormones for too long can lead to diseases and illnesses that require constant (or even lifelong) attention.

Headaches

A decrease in your blood sugar level and the release of stress hormones by your brain—due to going without food—are possible causes of headaches during the fasting window. Problems may also be a clear message from your body telling you that you are very low on water and getting dehydrated. It may happen if you are completely engrossed in your daily activities and forget to drink the required amount of water during your fasting.

To handle headaches, ensure you stay well hydrated throughout your fasting window. Keep in mind that exceeding the required amount of water per day may also result in adverse effects. Reducing your stress level can also keep headaches away.

Cravings

During your fasting periods, you might find that you have higher-than-usual levels of desire. It often happens because you tell yourself that you cannot have any food, so suddenly, you start craving many different foods. It is because all you are thinking about is food. As you think about food, you will begin to think about the different types of food you like and want. Then the cravings start.

You may also find yourself craving more sweets or carbs early on because your body is searching for an energy hit through glucose. While you do not want to have excessive sugar levels during your eating window, as this is bad for blood sugar, you can always have some. The ability to satisfy your cravings is one of the benefits of eating a diet that is not as restrictive as other foods.

Low Energy

A feeling of lethargy is not uncommon during fasting, especially at the start. It is your body's natural reaction to switching its source of energy from glucose in your meals to fat stored in your body. So, expect to feel a little less energized in your first few weeks of starting with intermittent fasting. To troubleshoot the feeling of lethargy, try as much as possible to stay away from overly strenuous activities. Keep things low-key. Spending more time sleeping or just relaxing is another right way to ensure that your energy reserves are not depleted too quickly. The first few weeks are not the time to test your limits or push yourself.

Foul Mood

You may find yourself being on edge during fasting, even if you are someone who is naturally predisposed to being good-natured. The reason for the feeling of edginess is straightforward. You are hungry, yet you won't eat, and you are struggling to keep your cravings in check; plus, you may already be feeling tired and sluggish. Add all of these to the internal hormone changes due to the sharp decline in your blood sugar levels, and it's no wonder why you may be in such a foul mood. Tempers can easily flare up, and you may be quick to become irritated. It is normal when beginning a fasting lifestyle.

Excess Urination

Fasting tends to make you visit the bathroom more frequently than usual. It is an expected side effect since you are drinking more water and other liquids than before. Avoiding water to reduce the number of times you use the bathroom is not a good idea at all, no matter how you look at it. Cutting down water intake while you are fasting will make your body become dehydrated very quickly. If that happens, losing weight will be the least of your problems. Whatever you do, do not avoid drinking water when you are fasting. Doing that is paving the way for a humongous health disaster waiting to happen. You don't want to do that.

Heartburn, Bloating, and Constipation

Your stomach is responsible for producing stomach acid, which is used to break down food and trigger the digestion process. When you eat substantial meals regularly, your body gets used to producing high amounts of stomach acid. As you transition to a fasting diet, your stomach has to get used to not making as much stomach acid.

You might also notice an increase in constipation and bloating. People who eat regularly consume high amounts of fiber and proteins that support a healthy digestion process. When you switch to the intermittent fasting cycle, you can still eat high-fiber and high-protein food; however, early on, you might find that you forget to do that. As you discover the right eating habits that work for you, it may take you some time to get used to finding ways to work in enough fiber and protein to keep your digestion flowing.

Heartburn may not be a widespread adverse effect, but it does sometimes occur in some individuals. Your stomach produces highly concentrated acids to help break down the foods you consume. When fasting, there is no food in your stomach to be broken down, even though acids have already been produced for that purpose. It may lead to heartburn.

Bloating goes hand in hand and can be very discomforting to individuals who suffer from it due to fasting.

Heeding the advice to drink adequate amounts of water usually keeps bloating and constipation in check. Heartburn typically resolves itself quickly, but you can take an antacid tablet or 2 if it persists. You may also consider eating fewer spicy foods when you break your fast.

You Might Experience Low Energy and Irritability

Until now, your body has been used to having a constant stream of energy pouring in all day long. From the time you wake up until you go to bed, your body receives energy from the foods you eat. So, when you stop eating regularly, your body grows confused. It has learned to create its energy rather than rely on the heat being offered to it by the food you are eating.

Depending on how you're eating, your body may also be growing used to consuming fat as a fuel source, rather than carbohydrates. It means that, in addition to losing its primary energy source, the body also has to switch how it consumes energy and where it gets that energy from. And all that can lead to a low point for a while.

Do things that exert the least amount of energy. If you regularly exercise and work out, reducing the amount of time you work out or switching to a more relaxed one like yoga can help you during the transition period.

You Might Start Feeling Cold

As you begin to adjust to your intermittent fasting diet, you might find that your fingers and toes get quite cold. It happens because blood flow towards your fat stores increases, so blood flow to your extremities reduces slightly. It supports your body in moving fat to your muscles so that it can be burned as fuel to keep your energy levels up.

You Might Find Yourself Overeating

The chances for overeating during the break of the fast are high, especially for beginners. Understandably, you will feel starving after going without food for longer than you used to. This hunger causes some people to eat hurriedly and surpass their standard meal size and average caloric intake. For others, overeating may be a result of an uncontrollable appetite. Hunger may push some people to prepare too much food for breaking their fast, and if they don't have a grip on their desire for food, they will continue to eat even when they are satiated. Overeating or binging when you break your fast will make it difficult to reach your optimal health and fitness goals.

Hunger Pangs

People who start intermittent fasting may initially feel quite hungry. It is a given if you are the type of person who tends to eat regular meals daily.

If you start feeling hungry, you can choose to wait it out if you have an eating window right around the corner. However, if there is a more extended waiting period or you feel starving, you should eat. Feeling hungry to the point that it becomes uncomfortable or distracting is not helpful and will not support you in successfully taking on the intermittent fasting diet. It is a pronounced side effect of going without food for longer than accustomed.

CHAPTER 5: INTERMITTENT FASTING SUCCESS STORIES

Look to those who have treaded before you. These stories are from real women who have lost weight using intermittent fasting. Most people who try this way of eating are pleased with their results. Some people are mad because they cannot lose weight rapidly, but they have no results because they eat mountains of food in their eating windows. The ones who do it right obtain inspirational successes.

Amanda's Fasting Story

I'm not sure where I first heard about IF. Probably some celebrity inspired me. Generally, I hate diets, and I would never have undergone this type of nutritional restriction. I believe in enjoying life and eating when you want to. But I had several health problems, including being overweight. I was 30 pounds overweight.

I read that you should go for 10 to 20 hours without eating. So, I chose to go 16 hours without eating as an excellent middle ground. Thus, I eat at 5 p.m. and then go to bed and have breakfast at eight. It's worked for me.

But I will tell you what was so hard. The hard part was not eating a nighttime meal. I had to get over that and just sip hot chicory tea. That's a lifesaver, by the way. I love chicory tea. I miss milk, but I use tea and water to fill the 15–16 fasting hours. I keep myself busy and sleep like a baby. It helped me get over the need to snack before bed. Now, I enjoy my meals so much more. They are not a routine or chore to fix, but a pleasure to look forward to.

I loved how adjustable it is, too. One time I had a late office dinner. Easy enough, I just switched breakfast to be at 11 a.m. It works seamlessly with your schedule. Just keep on top of the hours, and you're right.

During my first month, I dropped 10 pounds. Whoo-hoo! It showed right away. People kept giving me compliments. I didn't mean for these excellent results; they just happened. I didn't have any food restrictions, and I didn't hate my life. I just had to watch it when I ate. That's all.

The minute I get full, I don't want to eat anymore. I eat in the morning, but I usually don't want to; I chew to get my calories. I have lost edema in most of my body, and my blood pressure is normal. I sleep better because of the chicory, too. I have no more constipation or stomach pain. I recommend this approach for everyone, and I think everyone should adhere to it as much as possible. It's a great program that works with your body.

Ellice's Fasting Story

I had pretty much given up on remission from rheumatoid arthritis after giving birth. I was on the verge of despair, both physically and mentally. My quality of life was so low. Drug treatments don't work well for me, and my family has a long history of type I diabetes. I knew that I would develop diabetes because of the sudden jumps my pancreas was doing. I knew that something was wrong. I would break out in cold sweats and then feel terrible weakness until I ate. I didn't know what to do, and my options seemed nonexistent.

But on some baby board, I found some women raving about IF. Well, why not try it? Nothing else was working.

Recently, I made it 36 hours! I noticed that after starting this practice; I felt way better in the mornings. Usually, I hurt the worst in my joints at this time, so the pain was subsiding. One day, about a week on the diet, I woke up feeling light, like my depression had lifted. Then I realized that I hadn't eaten at 4 p.m. the day before. I was distracted and forgot about supper. I guess that happens, but it showed me that I don't need 3 meals a day, as they say.

A light bulb went off. If I didn't have so much protein in my body from dinner, maybe my body could not spare so much for autoimmune processes. Or maybe if my organs were resting and not moving so much with digestion, they did not make so many different movements and enzymes. Maybe my body was getting rid of toxins. Perhaps this approach was the secret to getting well from my RA (rheumatoid arthritis).

Now I do IF and restrict my solid food, but I drink all the water I want. Over 3 months, my condition has improved a lot; I'm a lot more flexible, and I have no more reflux esophagitis!

The only bad thing is that I have to stick with this for life. I broke my regimen once, and my symptoms flared up like clockwork. The elders knew something when they said not to eat after 6!

Jane's Fasting Story

A bit about me: I hit 210 pounds (I'm 5' 6" tall and 28 years old, so yeah, I was obese), and I hated looking at myself in photos or the mirror. I was humiliated by the scale in the doctor's office.

I tried a bunch of diets—even 'keto.' I couldn't follow them long enough to see long-term results. My friend said I was losing mostly water weight. I decided to try IF at her suggestion, fasting 16:8. So, I eat between 9 a.m. and 5 p.m., and then I don't eat from 5 p.m. to 9 a.m.. This schedule works since I go to work at 10 to grab breakfast and feel fulfilled as I work.

The weight loss has been slow but—a minus for IF—is still weight loss, and it's healthier than starving yourself. I believe you should lose no more than 10 pounds per month and that's what I've been doing. I'm glad I tried this approach, and I recommend it to anyone.

Melissa's Fasting Story

Intermittent fasting was perfect for me since I have problems with breakfast. I chose to eat from 12–8 and not eat from 8–12—I barely notice that I'm fasting since I'm mostly asleep then. I have lost 7 pounds in a month, just sleeping when I don't eat. It's effortless. No diet to follow, either.

The only minus is that sometimes I can't meet my caloric intake. I just don't have time. I am using Fat Secret and trying to meet my quota.

Candace's Fasting Story

I was 50 pounds overweight and then I got the worst news: My cholesterol was high, and my fasting blood sugar was 190. The idea of losing everything to diabetes scared me, so I knew I needed to change. I looked into diets ideal for prediabetics, and something about intermittent fasting came up. I looked into it more and decided to start.

No lie, it was not easy. I am used to getting up throughout the night to snack. My favorite hobby is relaxing at home with my husband and eating lots of snacks, too. And we love to go out and eat whenever we're hungry. I had to learn a lot of discipline and control. I started by not eating for 16 hours and didn't think I could do it. I tried eating a teaspoon of almond butter and drinking water when I felt hungry, and that helped.

Well, now I'm 8 pounds from my goal weight, meaning I've lost 42 pounds in the past 6 months. My cholesterol is better, and my doctor says I am no longer prediabetic. Plus, I feel better. I have more time and energy to play with my little boy and my husband. Our sex life is so much better. He has lost weight doing this plan with me, too, and we are glad.

CHAPTER 6: COMMON SIDE EFFECTS OF INTERMITTENT FASTING

Before I go into more details, you should pat yourself on the back for getting this far! If you've been doing intermittent fasting for some time now (or even if you've just started), you may have already experienced some common side effects. The good news is that, for most, the side effects are few and far between, and tend to disappear quickly once your body adapts to your new style of eating.

Fatigue or Brain Fog

Since most people choose to do their fast in the mornings, it's not uncommon to experience a bit of the old brain fog in the mornings, especially midmorning near the end of the fast. You'll undoubtedly know if you are experiencing any of these symptoms, and it's not ideal, especially if you have a job to do. Plus, you cannot afford to be making any silly mistakes on the job! Experiencing this in the first few days or up to 1 week of fasting is perfectly normal as your body adjusts; however, if this persists, then you've got a problem. Most commonly, this could be since you aren't eating enough during your eating window, or you only aren't receiving sufficient macronutrients.

The best way to combat is to make sure that you consume vitamins such as magnesium, iron, and vitamins (B, C, D, and E) to supplement your diet.

Additionally, make sure that you are eating enough complex carbs and protein. Try adding some more of these to your meal when you eat and see if this makes a difference.

If you are still experiencing brain fog and fatigue despite all this, persistently, it may be due to something else. As mentioned earlier, when intermittent fasting is done correctly, it can have extremely positive effects on the brain and general well-being.

Hair Loss

Please do not panic after reading this! I promise you that this is a doubtful side effect of IF. If you notice that you are losing more hair than average, it's unlikely for that problem to be due to your fasting but rather to a lack of nutrients. Referring back to the first point on the list, making sure you are taking your vitamins regularly and eating balanced meals during your eating window should prevent this from happening. Later in this book, I will dive deeper into how you can track and make sure you're getting the right number of calories and macronutrients for your body, so you don't have to worry about any adverse side effects. If you experience hair loss, it may be a good idea to visit your doctor and get to the bottom of this!

Menstrual Cycle Irregularities

Suppose you usually have a relatively regular menstrual cycle yet suddenly notice that you have missed a period or it's late. In that case, this could be a sign that your body is not receiving enough calories (or you're pregnant)! Another term for this is amenorrhea, which is a clear symptom of starvation or being underweight, and it causes concern.

Constipation

Remember, I mentioned earlier the importance of hydration? Only drinking enough water throughout the day will prevent constipation. This side effect is much more common in women who forget to drink water during their fast, which is bound to cause some severe stomach issues regardless. Drink your H20, and you'll be good to go! Another great way to avoid or treat constipation is to ensure that you are getting adequate fiber in your diet. Merely incorporating whole grains into your next meal—such as whole wheat bread, oats, and quinoa—can help in getting things moving in your bowels.

Additionally, some people find that by simply changing their environment, diet, or general lifestyle, they notice a change in their bowel movements as their body grows to adjust. It is perfectly normal and certainly not a cause for concern. If the problem persists after 1 week while still drinking plenty of water and sticking to a routine, then it is recommended that you head to see your doctor.

Disturbed Sleep

I have never experienced this side effect while following IF, but studies have linked IF with disturbed sleep. The studies suggested that fasting during the day affects negatively the REM (rapid eye movement) sleep stages by reducing it. It isn't great news, as REM enhances memory, concentration, and overall better mental processing (Almeneessier & BaHammam, 2018). With that being said, many women have claimed that they slept better while practicing intermittent fasting.

Regardless, everyone is different. If you do find that you are not sleeping and usually do, then it may be time to consult your doctor to determine the underlying issue.

Changes in Mood

Restricting your food intake in any way is bound to make most women a little grumpy, or "hangry," as the saying goes! It is perfectly normal, especially in the beginning stages of your fast. With that being said, if you are finding that IF is severely influencing your life, your work, or your relationships, then it may be time to decide if this is worth your time. The best way to determine is to try IF for 1 week or 2 weeks. If you are still feeling really awful, then this may be an indicator to stop, so instead, consult a dietician with regards to a new diet plan ("If you have any of these intermittent fasting side effects, it might mean it isn't a great fit for you," 2021).

I can personally vouch for mood changes, but the good news is that they are not permanent, and you can talk yourself out of them with the right mindset and a positive attitude. There is no better feeling in my personal experience than looking at the clock and seeing "noon," knowing you have completed your fast successfully! Plus, that first morsel of food tastes even better. The more successful fasts you can achieve, the more your body will become accustomed to them, and going without food will become more and more comfortable. You'll see!

Low Blood Sugar

If you're anything like me, a low blood sugar level is something that hits me like a bus, especially when I haven't eaten anything decent all day! If you have a low blood sugar level, chances are your body will let you know!

44

Common signs of low blood sugar levels include headaches, feeling lightheaded and weak, and shaking or nausea. If you experience any of these side effects, then it's time to eat something like stat! If you have diabetes, you should not fast for long periods, as this can wreak havoc on your blood sugar and become a dangerous situation. Rather be safe than sorry!

CHAPTER 7: RECIPES

1.   Healthy Breakfast Smoothie

Preparation Time: 5 minutes

Cooking Time: 1 minute

Servings: 1

Ingredients:

- 1 ¼ cups coconut milk, or almond or regular dairy milk
- ½ cup kale or spinach, or both (¼ cup each) if you prefer
- ½ avocado, sliced into smaller pieces
- ¾ cup cucumber, cut into smaller pieces
- 1 cup green grapes
- ¼ tsp. ginger, peeled and grated
- 1 scoop plant-based protein powder
- Honey, to taste

Directions:

1. Orderly, mix all the ingredients in a small bowl.
2. Blend them until the mixture is smooth.
3. Taste the mixture and add as much honey as you desire.
4. Pour into a glass and serve.

Nutrition:

- Calories: 117
- Fats: 15 g
- Protein: 20 g

2. Avocado-Egg Bowls

Preparation Time: 10 minutes

Cooking Time: 40 minutes

Servings: 3

Ingredients:

- 1 tsp. coconut oil
- 2 organic eggs, free-range
- Salt and pepper, to sprinkle
- 1 avocado, large and ripe

For Garnishing:

- Chopped walnuts, as many as you like
- Balsamic pearls to taste
- Fresh thyme to taste

Directions:

1. Slice the avocado in 2, then take out the pit and remove enough of the inside so that there is enough space inside to accommodate an entire egg.
2. Cut off a little bit of the bottom of the avocado so that the avocado will sit upright as you place it on a stable surface.

3. Open the eggs and put each of the yolks in a separate bowl or container. Place the egg whites in the same small bowl. Sprinkle some pepper and salt into the whites according to your taste, then mix them well.

4. Melt the coconut oil in a pan that has a lid that fits, and place it over medium-high heat.

5. Put the avocado 'boats' meaty-side down and skin-side up in the pan, and sauté them for approx. 35 seconds, or when they become darker.

6. Turn them over, then add to the spaces inside, almost filling the inside with the egg whites.

7. Then lower the temperature and cover the pan. Let them sit covered for approx. 16–20 minutes, or until the whites are just about fully cooked.

8. Gently, add 1 yolk onto each of the avocados and keep cooking them for 4–5 minutes, or just until they get to the point of cooking you want them to.

9. Move the avocados to a dish and add toppings to each of them using the walnuts, the balsamic pearls, or/and thyme.

Nutrition:

- Calories: 215
- Fats: 18 g
- Protein: 9 g

3.   Blueberries Breakfast Bowl

Preparation Time: 35 minutes

Cooking Time: 0 minutes

Servings: 1

Ingredients:

- 1 tsp. chia seed
- 1 cup almond milk
- ¼ cup fresh blueberries or fresh fruits

Directions:

1. Mix the chia seeds with almond milk. Stir periodically.
2. Put in the fridge to cool and serve with the blueberries or fresh fruit. Enjoy!

Nutrition:

- Calories: 202
- Fats: 16.8 g
- Protein: 10.2 g

4. <u>Feta-Filled Tomato-Topped Oldie Omelet</u>

Preparation Time: 5 minutes

Cooking Time: 6 minutes

Servings: 1

Ingredients:

- 1 tbsp. coconut oil
- 2 eggs
- 1 ½ tbsp. milk
- A dash salt and pepper
- ¼ cup tomatoes, sliced into cubes
- 2 tbsp. feta cheese, crumbled

Directions:

1. Beat the eggs with pepper, salt, milk, and the remaining spices.
2. Pour the mixture along with coconut oil into a preheated pan.
3. Stir in the tomatoes and cheese. Cook for 6 minutes, or until the cheese melts.

Nutrition:

- Calories: 335
- Fats: 28.4 g
- Protein: 16.2 g

5.   Carrot Breakfast Salad

Cooking Time: 4 hours

Preparation Time: 5 minutes

Servings: 4

Ingredients:

- 2 tbsp. olive oil
- 2 lbs. baby carrots, peeled and halved
- 3 garlic cloves, minced
- 2 yellow onions, chopped
- ½ cup vegetable stock
- ⅓ cup tomatoes, crushed
- A pinch salt and black pepper

Directions:

1. In your slow cooker, combine all the ingredients, cover, and cook on high for 4 hours.
2. Divide into bowls and serve for breakfast.

Nutrition:

- Calories: 437
- Protein: 2.39 g
- Fats: 39.14 g

6.   Paprika Lamb Chops

Preparation Time: 10 minutes

Cooking Time: 15 minutes

Servings: 4

Ingredients:

- 2 lamb racks, cut into chops
- Salt and pepper, to taste
- 3 tbsp. paprika
- ¾ cup cumin powder
- 1 tsp. chili powder

Directions:

1 . Take a bowl and add the paprika, cumin, chili, salt, pepper, and stir.
2 . Add the lamb chops and rub the mixture.
3 . Heat grill over medium heat, add the lamb chops and cook for 5 minutes.
4 . Flip the lamb chops over and cook for 5 minutes more, then flip again.
5 . Cook for 2 minutes, flip, and cook for 2 minutes more. Serve and enjoy.

Nutrition:

- Calories: 200
- Fats: 5 g
- Protein: 8 g

7. <u>Delicious Turkey Wrap</u>

Preparation Time: 10 minutes

Cooking Time: 10 minutes

Servings: 6

Ingredients:

- 1 ¼ lb. ground turkey, lean
- 4 green onions, minced
- 1 tbsp. olive oil
- 1 garlic clove, minced
- 2 tsp. chili paste
- 8 oz. water chestnut, diced
- 3 tbsp. hoisin sauce
- 2 tbsp. coconut amino
- 1 tbsp. rice vinegar
- 12 butter lettuce leaves
- ⅛ tsp. salt

Directions:

1 . Take a pan and place it over medium heat, then add the turkey, and garlic to the pan.
2 . Heat for 6 minutes, or until cooked.
3 . Transfer the turkey to a bowl.

4 . Add the onions and water chestnuts.

5 . Stir in the hoisin sauce, coconut amino, rice vinegar, and chili paste.

6 . Toss well and transfer the mix to the lettuce leaves. Serve and enjoy.

Nutrition:

- Calories: 162

- Fats: 4 g

- Protein: 23 g

8.   Bacon & Chicken Garlic Wrap

Preparation Time: 15 minutes

Cooking Time: 10 minutes

Servings: 4

Ingredients:

- 1 chicken fillet, cut into small cubes
- 8–9 bacon slices, thinly cut to fit the cubes
- 6 garlic cloves, minced

Directions:

1. Preheat your oven to 400°F.
2. Line a baking tray with aluminum foil.
3. Add the minced garlic to a bowl and rub each chicken piece with it.
4. Wrap a bacon piece around each garlic chicken bite.
5. Secure each bite with a toothpick.
6. Transfer the bites to the baking sheet, keeping a little bit of space between them.
7. Bake for about 15–20 minutes, or until crispy. Serve and enjoy.

Nutrition:

- Calories: 260
- Fats: 19 g
- Protein: 22 g

9. Pumpkin Pancakes

Preparation Time: 10 minutes

Cooking Time: 15 minutes

Servings: 6

Ingredients:

- 3 eggs, large, and egg whites separated
- ⅔ cups organic oats
- 6 oz. pumpkin purée
- 1 scoop collagen peptides
- 1 tsp. stevia powder
- ½ tsp. cinnamon
- Cooking spray, as needed
- Fruits, optional

Directions:

1 . Combine and blend all the ingredients in a blender and mix well.
2 . Apply the cooking spray to the pan to coat it properly.
3 . Pour some of the batter into the pan to coat the pan properly.
4 . Wait till the edges of the pancake brown up a little bit.
5 . Flip the pancake over and cook from the other side.
6 . You can serve it with fruits.

Nutrition:

- Calories: 70
- Fats: 3 g
- Protein: 3 g

10. Cherry Smoothie Bowl

Preparation Time: 15 minutes

Cooking Time: 0 minute

Servings: 1

Ingredients:

- ½ cup organic rolled oats
- ½ cup almond milk, unsweetened
- 1 tbsp. chia seeds
- 1 tsp. hemp seeds
- 2 tsp. almonds, sliced
- 1 tbsp. almond butter
- 1 tsp. vanilla extract
- ½ cup berries, fresh
- 1 cup cherries, frozen
- 1 cup plain Greek yogurt

Directions:

1. Soak the organic rolled oats in almond milk.
1. Prepare a smooth blend with the soaked oats, frozen cherries, yogurt, chia seeds, almond butter, and vanilla extract. Pour the mixture into 2 bowls.

2 . To each bowl, add equal parts of the hemp seeds, sliced almonds, and fresh cherries.

Nutrition:

- Calories: 130
- Fats: 0 g
- Protein: 1 g

11. Kale & Sausage Omelet

Preparation Time: 10 minutes

Cooking Time: 10 minutes

Servings: 2

Ingredients:

- 4 eggs
- 2 cups kale, chopped
- 4 oz. sausages, sliced
- 4 tbsp. ricotta cheese
- 6 oz. roasted squash
- 2 tbsp. olive oil
- Salt and black pepper, to taste
- Fresh parsley, for garnishing

Directions:

1. In a medium-sized bowl, blend the eggs, salt, and pepper. Then whisk in the kale and the ricotta cheese. In another bowl, mash the squash.
2. Add the squash to the egg mixture. In a pan over medium heat, heat 1 tablespoon of olive oil and cook the sausages for 5 minutes. Drizzle the remaining olive oil.

3 . Pour the egg mixture over and cook for 2 minutes on both sides. With a spatula, run around the edges of the omelet and slide it onto a platter. Serve topped with parsley.

Nutrition:

- Calories: 258
- Fats: 22 g
- Protein: 12 g

12. <u>Sausage Quiche with Tomatoes</u>

Preparation Time: 15 minutes

Cooking Time: 10 minutes

Servings: 6

Ingredients:

- 6 eggs
- 12 oz. raw sausage rolls
- 10 cherry tomatoes halved
- 2 tbsp. heavy cream
- 2 tbsp. Parmesan, grated
- Salt and black pepper, to taste
- 2 tbsp. parsley, chopped
- 5 eggplant slices

Directions:

1. Preheat the oven to 370°F. Press the sausage rolls onto the bottom of a greased pie dish. On top of the sausage, carefully arrange the eggplant slices.
2. Top with cherry tomatoes. Whisk together the eggs along with the heavy cream, Parmesan cheese, salt, and pepper.
3. Spoon the egg mixture over the sausage and bake for about 40 minutes. Serve with parsley.

Nutrition:

- Calories: 340
- Fats: 28 g
- Protein: 1.7 g

13. Bacon & Cream Cheese Mug Muffins

Preparation Time: 15 minutes

Cooking Time: 15 minutes

Servings: 2

Ingredients:

- ¼ cup Flaxseed Meal
- 1 egg
- 2 tbsp. heavy cream
- 2 tbsp. pesto
- ¼ cup almond flour
- ¼ tsp. baking soda
- Salt and black pepper, to taste
- 2 tbsp. cream cheese
- 4 bacon slices
- ½ medium avocado, sliced

Directions:

1. Mix the Flaxseed Meal, almond flour, and baking soda in a bowl. Add the egg, heavy cream, and pesto. Then whisk well. Season with salt and pepper.

2. Divide the mixture between 2 ramekins. Microwave for 60–90 seconds. Let cool slightly before filling.

3. Put the bacon in a nonstick skillet and cook until crispy, then set aside.

4. Transfer the muffins onto a plate and cut them in half crosswise. Assemble the sandwiches by spreading the cream cheese and topping with the bacon and avocado slices.

Nutrition:

- Calories: 511
- Fats: 38 g
- Protein: 16 g

14. Chorizo & Cheese Omelet

Preparation Time: 10 minutes

Cooking Time: 10 minutes

Servings: 2

Ingredients:

- 4 eggs, beaten
- 4 oz. mozzarella, grated
- 1 tbsp. butter
- 8 chorizo slices, thin
- 1 tomato, sliced
- Salt and black pepper to taste

Directions:

1. Whisk the eggs with salt and pepper.
2. In a cast-iron skillet, add the butter and cook the eggs for 30 seconds. Create a layer with the chorizo slices.
3. Arrange the sliced tomato and mozzarella over the chorizo and cook for about 3 minutes. Cover the skillet and continue cooking for 3 more minutes, or until the omelet is completely set.
4. With a spatula, run around the edges of the omelet and flip it onto a plate folded-side down. Serve.

Nutrition:

- Calories 451
- Fats: 36.5 g
- Protein: 30 g

CHAPTER 8: BENEFITS OF PLANNING

Meal planning is beneficial in many practical ways. One of its most significant benefits is on a person's health, mainly if it combines healthy balanced food and proper portion control.

Benefit # 1—It Helps Improve Your General Health

Whether or not you have a medical condition, meal planning can improve your overall health when the meals provide all the macro and micronutrients your body needs. It also enables you to avoid saturated fats and processed sugars, which most people would reach for if they're hungry and just want something satisfying.

Benefit # 2—It Ensures that You Can Eat on Time

Preparing your meals in advance helps manage hunger pains. Missing a meal or delaying it can cause your blood sugar level to drop too low, a condition otherwise known as hypoglycemia.

Hypoglycemia can cause shaking, disorientation, and irritability. You may even have a seizure if your blood sugar level gets any lower. Having your meal already prepared ensures that you can always eat on time and, therefore, decrease the risk of low blood sugar.

Benefit # 3—It Lowers Your Risk of Heart Disease

Diabetes increases the risk of heart disease. With the help of a dietician, planning your meals can help you reduce this risk. Because meal prep minimizes the time you need to spend in the kitchen, you'll have more opportunities to exercise and do other activities that promote a healthier lifestyle.

Benefit # 4—It Lowers Your Risk of Cancer

Diabetes also increases the risk of all forms of cancer. While experts are still unable to identify the exact link between these two conditions, cancer patients are advised to pursue a healthy lifestyle, including eating a balanced diet and getting adequate exercise. Because these activities are also encouraged among people with diabetes, the risk of cancer is lowered.

Benefit # 5—It Helps You Maintain Healthy Body Weight

Again, portion control plays a part in this area. Even if you eat healthy food, overindulging can lead to an unhealthy weight gain, making it harder to control your blood sugar level.

If left unchecked, this could lead to high blood sugar levels or hyperglycemia, which can cause various complications that include heart and liver damage and the loss of kidney function.

It's important to note that while meal planning can help keep the effects of diabetes under control, you and your dietician still need to conduct a periodic examination of its effectiveness and make changes whenever necessary.

Benefit#6—It Lowers Your Risk of Osteoporosis

This condition can affect both men and women. Your bones become weak, brittle, and easy to fracture as you get older. It is an especially significant issue among women who are most likely to experience complications due to this bone loss.

High blood sugar levels are believed to be the cause of the brittle bone disease known as osteoporosis. Once again, Diabetes can be managed with meal planning and other healthy lifestyle changes that prevent or delay its onset.

How to Do a Meal Planning—Meal Planning Approaches

There are usually 3 types of meal plans:

- The exchange meal plan

- Constant carbohydrate meal plan

- Carbohydrate counting meal plan

The Exchange Meal Plan: Foods are segregated into 6 groups in the exchange plan. There is meal planning flexibility by substituting or exchanging from the food lists. In other words, you can have something else from another group that has the same nutritional content. The exchange (serving) number from each group for each snack and meal should be based on how many calories you need every day.

It is a beneficial meal planning approach for those who have diabetes and are trying to lose weight, and also for those who have to keep a close watch on the nutrients and calories they take each day.

The two other approaches are also based on having a balanced diet. However, they focus mainly on matching the insulin or diabetes medication amount with the number of carbohydrates.

The Constant Carbohydrate Plan: According to this type of meal planning, you have to eat a set amount of carbohydrates in every snack and meal and then take the diabetes medication or insulin at the correct amount, and you have to watch out for blood sugar level spikes during the day. There is no flexibility in this meal plan, but it is a simple one for those whose physical activity levels and food intake stay relatively constant every day.

The Carbohydrate Counting Plan: This type of meal planning approach is about calculating the carbs in food consumed every day (both snacks and meals). The carb amount is then matched with the insulin dosage. It is the right approach for managing diabetes by an insulin dose packed in the meals. It gives more flexibility as you are taking insulin during the meals and not at the same time every day.

A dose of insulin will help, but only if you are on the right diabetic diet. No external support can help if you are not consuming the right foods in the correct amounts, and if you are not eating the right part at the right time.

Step-By-Step Guide to Diabetic Meal Planning

Select your meal planning method (from the ones mentioned above). You can also combine 2 methods based on your nutritional goals and lifestyle.

Maintain a Schedule: Plan your meals for the week on a particular day every week. Make sure that you shop for groceries and do your cooking before.

Plan Correctly: Calculate the right number of meals, including those when you are planning to eat out.

Recipes: Select different types of recipes so that you can keep your food interesting. There are plenty of options to choose from.

Grocery Shopping: Don't spend too much time shopping for groceries. Have a list ready before you go to the supermarket or buy online.

Reduce Your Kitchen Time: Have a plan for the meals you want to prepare first. You can plan this based on the cooking time needed.

Store: Refrigerate and store so that the food can be reused—also label the foods with the cooking date. Use the right containers for storing.

Reading Food Labels

It is always a great idea to read food labels carefully. Look at the ingredients, calories, and nutritional information. It will help you better know the foods you are eating.

Check the information on carbohydrates especially, because this can impact your blood sugar levels. You will find them listed on the food labels. The 2 main types of carbohydrates are starches and sugars. Sugar types include:

- Fructose (the sugar you get from some baked foods and fruits)
- Glucose (sugar within us, but you will also get this from foods, such as cookies, soft drinks, and cakes)
- Lactose (the sugar you get from yogurt and milk)
- Starches (from vegetables like peas, corn, potatoes, cereals, bread, and rice)

Remember, your body will break down or convert more of the carbohydrates into glucose, which will then be absorbed into your bloodstream. Your pancreas will release the insulin hormone when the level of glucose goes up. Insulin will move glucose into your cells, where it will be used as energy.

You must keep a tab on the carbs, no matter what meal plan you go with. It will make it easier for you to balance the carbohydrate intake, activity level, and insulin, as it will help you immensely in diabetes control.

Check the carbs amount and serving size to find out the carb intake in each serving. For instance:

- Serving size—120 milliliters (½ cup)
- Carbs in each serving—7 grams
- Food amount—240 milliliters (1 cup)
- Carbs—14 grams (2 servings of 7 grams each)

The Art of Storage

I have mentioned already that storing and reusing is a good idea. So, picking the right food storage containers will make a huge difference. Here are some contained recommendations that you will find useful:

- Keep your ready-to-cook ingredients in airtight containers. You can pick reusable, washable, stainless steel containers and silicone baggies. The food will stay fresh and crisp.

- BPA-free, microwave-safe containers are good for health and convenience. Select collapsible silicone or Pyrex® glassware containers.

- Freezer-safe containers are right because they limit the nutrient loss and freezer burns. Get wide-mount mason jars. But remember to keep a 2.5 cm or 1-inch space at the top as the food can expand when it is frozen.

- Compartmentalized, leak-proof containers like bento lunch boxes are suitable for meals and lunches where the ingredients are often mixed later on.

CHAPTER 9: INTERMITTENT FASTING FOOD LIST—HOW TO CHOOSE THE BEST FOODS

During intermittent fasting, feeding is more about being healthy than simply losing weight quickly. Thus, selecting nutrient-dense foods, such as veggies, fruits, lean proteins, and healthy fats is critically important.

The list of intermittent fasting foods should include:

Protein

0.8 grams of protein of your body is the RDA (recommended dietary allowance) for protein (or 20% of your daily calories). Depending on your health objectives, your requirements can differ.

By reducing energy consumption, increasing satiety, and improving metabolism, protein helps you lose weight. Besides, increased protein consumption helps in creating muscle when paired with strength training. As muscle burns more calories than fat, having more muscle in the body naturally increases the metabolism. A recent study indicates that in healthy men, having more muscle in the legs will help in reducing the development of belly fat.

The IF food list for protein includes:

Poultry and fish:

- Seafood

- Eggs

- Dairy products

- Beans and legumes

- Soy

- Seeds and nuts

- Whole grains

Carbs

45–65% of the daily calories should come from carbohydrates, according to the RDA for carbs. Carbs are the main source of your body's nutrition. The other 2 are fat and protein. Carbs come in different ways. Sugar, carbohydrate, and starch are the most notable among them.

Carbs for causing weight gain also get a poor score. Not all carbohydrates, however, are produced equally and are not necessarily fattening. The type and amount of carbs you eat depends on whether or not you can gain weight. Make sure that foods high in fiber and starch but low in sugar are selected. A 2015 study indicates that consuming 30 grams of fiber every day will lead to weight loss, glucose level increments, and blood pressure decreases. It isn't an uphill struggle to get 30 grams of fiber from your diet. You will get them by consuming a basic egg sandwich, Mediterranean barley with chickpeas, peanut butter apple, and enchiladas with chicken and black peas.

The IF food list for carbs includes:

- Sweet potatoes

- Quinoa

- Oats

- Beetroots

- Brown rice

- Mangoes

- Apples

- Berries

- Bananas

- Kidney beans

- Pears

- Carrots

- Broccoli

- Brussels sprouts

- Avocado

- Almonds

- Chickpeas

- Chia seeds

Fats

Fats should contribute 20–35% of your daily calories, according to RDA in 2015-2020. Most significantly, saturated fat does not account for more than 10% of daily calories—fats, depending on the form, maybe good, poor, or simply in-between. Trans fat, for example, increases inflammation, decreases good cholesterol levels, and increases bad cholesterol levels. They are found in fruit and baked goods that are fried.

Saturated fats can raise the risk of heart disease. Expert views on this, however, vary. Eating them in moderation is wise. High levels of saturated fats are present in red meat, whole milk, coconut oil, and baked goods. The monounsaturated and polyunsaturated fats provide healthy fats. These fats can reduce the risk of heart disease, decrease blood pressure, and decrease fat levels in the blood. The sources rich in fats include olive oil, peanut oil, canola oil, safflower oil, sunflower oil, and soybean oil.

The IF food list for fats includes:

- Avocados

- Cheese

- Nuts

- Whole eggs

- Dark chocolate

- Chia seeds

- Fatty fish

- Full-fat yogurt

- Extra virgin olive oil (EVOO)

For a Healthy Gut

An increasing body of evidence suggests that the secret to overall well-being is intestinal health. Your intestine has billions of bacteria known as microbiota in its home.

These bacteria impair your gut health, digestion, and mental health. They can also play a critical role in many chronic disorders. Therefore, particularly when you are fasting intermittently, you should take care of those tiny bugs in your stomach.

The intermittent fasting food list for a healthy gut include:

- All vegetables
- Kefir
- Fermented vegetables
- Kimchi
- Miso
- Sauerkraut
- Kombucha
- Tempeh

These foods will also help you lose weight, in addition to keeping your gut safe by…

- reducing fat absorption from the gut.
- increasing the excretion via stools of ingested fat.
- reducing the consumption of calories.

Hydration

The daily fluid requirements, according to the National Academies of Sciences, Engineering, and Medicine, are:

- About 3.7 liters (15 ½ cups) for men

- About 2.7 liters (11 ½ cups) for women

Fluids include water, as well as water-containing foods and beverages.

During intermittent fasting, keeping hydrated is important for your health. Headaches, extreme tiredness, and dizziness may be caused by dehydration. Dehydration can make these side effects of fasting worse, or even extreme if you are still dealing with them.

The intermittent fasting food list for hydration includes:

- Water
- Black coffee or tea
- Sparkling water
- Watermelon
- Cantaloupe
- Peaches
- Strawberries
- Oranges
- Lettuce
- Cucumber
- Skim milk
- Celery
- Plain yogurt
- Tomatoes

Interestingly, drinking a lot of water will help with weight loss as well as with decreasing appetite or consumption of food, and with speeding up the fat-burning processes.

CHAPTER 10: HOW TO STAY MOTIVATED

Find Support

The first weeks of intermittent fasting can be frustrating as well as damn hard. If you don't see any physical results, then it may prompt you to give up.

Many find it difficult to stay motivated, but the tips below will help you stay motivated throughout the journey.

First, it is easier to stay on track when there is support. This could be your husband, best friend, or another family member. Sit down with them and explain the basics of the chosen intermittent fasting method.

Be supportive of each other on days when some of you don't feel like starving or exercising. It will be more fun if you can plan meals, buy groceries, exercise, and study with someone.

If you have someone interested in your success, you don't want to do anything to let them down.

Set Achievable Goals

It's best to start with short-term goals—knowing you can achieve them will make it easier for you. Every goal achieved must be followed by a reward. But it doesn't have to be junk food.

The term for achieving the goal can be different—a couple of days or a week. For example, stick to the crescendo method for a week. Be sure to write down the goal and achievement reward.

Get a massage or buy new sportswear. This will boost your momentum and motivation.

At the initial stage, the slogan of Alcoholics Anonymous will help you: "One day at a time!" This means that you will fast only today and not worry about what happens tomorrow.

Over time, you can move on to more serious long-term goals.

Keep a Journal

This is a great way to test the positive changes that have occurred since you started fasting. Keep a journal and start writing down how you are feeling and your progress.

It's important to take the time to assess the changes in your body and life. See if your clothes are right for you, how much energy you now have to play with your children, and if your sleep has improved.

Track your positive progress and write in a journal every time you feel a lack of motivation.

Also, the journal will ease your psycho-emotional state. Once you start writing down your experiences, consider that it goes away and no longer concerns you. This will cleanse you emotionally.

Use this method every time you feel bad. It is self-tested and works!

Don't Scold Yourself

Yes, there are days when you give up and succumb to temptation, like eating a cookie or two. But this is not a reason to scold yourself. You need to be compassionate, including towards yourself.

Don't start talking negatively about yourself just because you ate something you shouldn't have. It is important to accept what has been done and continue moving forward.

There is a risk of starting a process called a vicious circle. You make a mistake, then scold yourself, get nervous about it, eat something harmful, and scold yourself again.

In this case, it is very important to find something to praise yourself for and stop on time.

Pray or Meditate

When you feel like you're losing motivation, take some time for yourself. There are many ways to strengthen your soul and spirit. This can be prayer, scripture reading, or meditation.

It will help you love yourself, even as difficulties come your way.

Focus on the Good

I bet you have increased energy levels in the first few weeks. This is especially noticeable after the feeding phase. You became more focused, euphoric, and even creative. It's great!

Most likely, you have more downtime, especially if this is the fasting phase. You used to spend it on cooking, but now you can use it as you wish.

Even if you do not notice noticeable weight loss in the first days and weeks of intermittent fasting, there are always positive points. They should be your main focus.

Think about the extra time you can now spend with your family and loved ones, and all the extra activities, motivation, and energy. Don't expect quick results, but stick to your goal.

Fat burning usually becomes noticeable after the third or fourth week. Furthermore, it will be stable.

Slow Down

The success of your diet depends on changes in your lifestyle. These changes take time and do not occur in 1 minute/day/week. If you want to lose weight and remain fit, then you need to lose weight slowly.

You can starve yourself and lose a few pounds, but it won't do any good. The more gradual and stable weight loss is, the easier it is to maintain it. Intermittent fasting is a great diet option that produces lasting results.

Make sure you progress smoothly. You should not rush, and the results will definitely appear.

Be Your Personal Coach

You are the main motivator. You can program your mind to only think in the right direction. You need to manage yourself, evaluate your efforts positively, and be constantly reminded of your motivation.

Look at yourself in the mirror and tell your reflection (out loud) that you can overcome food cravings. Remember, IF is the path to great health.

You can program your mind and body this way every day. After that, your body will become an incredibly fat-burning machine. When you use these self-motivating techniques, your brain will believe whatever you tell yourself.

If you think you will fail, you will inevitably fail. But if you truly believe that you will succeed, you will!

Failure Is Normal

The temptation may arise, and there will be times when you succumb to it. There is nothing wrong with that, and it is allowed from time to time. After all, you are only human.

It's okay to face failure, but don't take it as if you were a failure. Your attitude towards those moments of weakness can reinvigorate you as you work towards the desired results.

The important thing is not that you can fall, but that you rise and move on!

Don't Be a Perfectionist

What would you do if you couldn't resist the Oreo® cookies? Perfectionist thinking hinders success more than any other factor. If the 200-calorie relief is just a 'concession' and nothing more, then it's okay. However, if for you it is like a failure and an excuse to quit, then it can lead to a loss of 1,000 calories.

Patience Is a Great Workout

A significant obstacle to dieting is the weight loss plateau. You can eat right and exercise, but the numbers on the scale will not change.

This is known as a weight loss plateau and has been experienced by every dieter. Just stop and congratulate yourself on your success. This is part of the weight loss process.

Forgive Yourself

Remember, intermittent fasting is not a walk in the park. Once you start practicing, you will realize that it is not as easy as it seems at first glance.

There are times when you go astray. You may have gone to your birthday and ate a delicious meal, even though you were supposed to be fasting. This is normal, and you don't have to blame yourself for it.

Don't berate yourself for being human. Instead of punishing yourself, recognize the mistake, start over, and keep moving forward.

Reward Yourself

Fasting and eating properly require some effort. At times, you can get bored with it and want to give up. Therefore, it is very important to reward yourself for achieving a goal. The goal can be large or small. It could be something as simple as having sweet treats during the day. When you reach your goal, indulge in something.

The reward doesn't have to be extravagant. Perhaps you could buy that new dress you've been eyeing. The reward should not be food-related.

Therefore, if you lost 5 pounds in 10 days, rewarding yourself with a pint of ice cream is clearly not worth it. It doesn't make any sense.

When you celebrate your success, it changes the way you feel about yourself and your diet. It will also provide additional stimulation—you will keep working towards your goal even when you want to give up.

Keeping Motivated

Keeping motivated throughout the intermittent fasting journey can be difficult. There are many situations when you want to give up everything. At such moments, you need to remember why you started to practice IF, and why it should be continued further.

Yes, failures can happen. But this is not a reason to scold yourself or give up everything. You should not scold yourself even if you do not see any results yet. If you do everything right, they will definitely be there. You just need to be patient and wait a bit.

CHAPTER 11: POSSIBLE CHALLENGES WITH INTERMITTENT FASTING

Nothing in the world is perfect. That being said, the "eat-stop-eat" protocol has its share of potential challenges or negative side effects. These include the following:

Impaired Physical Performance

Particularly during your fasting moments, intermittent fasting may reduce your physical strength as a result of a lack of calories from food. This is because energy from food is the easiest to process or access for physical performance compared to body fat. Relying on body fat for energy when it comes to situations where optimal physical performance is crucial, such as sports competitions or when working out, may cause you to perform below optimal levels.

And when you're working out, suboptimal efforts can keep you from optimizing your body's ability to produce human growth hormone and replenish your glycogen stores immediately after working out. When this happens, your risks of muscle catabolism become high. That's why it's crucial that you synchronize the time of your exercise/workouts with your eating window. That will increase your chances of optimal efforts in the gym and reduce your risks of muscle catabolism.

Potential Eating Disorders

Despite the lack of documented studies, dieticians can attest that it is possible to develop eating disorders when fasting intermittently. In particular, many intermittent fasters tend to overcompensate during their eating windows to the point that they are regularly overeating or worse, binge-eating as they break their fasts. And oftentimes, this happens with unhealthy foods that are highly processed and high in refined sugars and trans fats, which are 2 of the deadliest ingredients that we can find in many commercially available processed foods.

That's why if you're at risk of or are already suffering from an eating disorder, it's best to stay off intermittent fasting. You might aggravate your condition or cause yourself to acquire an eating disorder if you fast regularly.

Sterility

Without a shadow of a doubt, reproductive health is highly dependent on getting the right nutrients at the right amounts; for example, adequate calories. An example of this is amenorrhea, which refers to the loss or cessation of a woman's menstrual cycle. This condition has been linked to low body weight and not eating enough.

The exact reasons for this relationship aren't strongly established because human IF trials weren't large enough to make certain conclusions. But in one study on female rats, intermittent fasting was shown to obstruct the subjects' fertility.

Sustainability

Regardless of what the staunchest IF fanatic says, fasting isn't the norm. Humans are wired to eat, so when given opportunities to do so, people would grab them (the foods). The only reason why fasting frequently was 'natural' thousands of years ago was because of a lack of food, which our early ancestors had no control over. In short, they 'fasted' against their will.

That being said, it may not be realistic for the majority of the human race to fast intermittently for the rest of their lives. Yes, it's possible for some people with extreme levels of self-control and self-discipline to sustain IF over the long haul, but they're the exceptions rather than the norm. It's no different from the fact that millions of people all over the world play basketball but only a handful can ever make a serious living out of it, regardless of how hard they work at their games.

Now, it doesn't mean you shouldn't fast intermittently. What I'm saying is that it can be very challenging to sustain it over the long haul, and if you set your eyes on the long term from the get-go, you might get very disappointed and quit early on. The key to making IF work for you is to take baby steps. What does that look like?

In terms of following the eat-stop-eat protocol, for example, instead of starting your first fasting days with a full 24-hour fast, start by delaying your breakfast as long as you possibly can. Why?

Believe it or not, you're already fasting intermittently without you knowing it. You do this when you sleep at night, assuming you don't wake up for midnight snacks. So, if you get an average of 8 hours of nightly sleep, this means you're already fasting 8 hours every day.

When you delay eating breakfast, you add to that number of hours you fasted overnight. That's why it's more realistic to start this way; for example, eating 1 hour or 2 after waking up. Then gradually move up your breakfast until it becomes brunch, and delay it further over the next few weeks or months until you're able to fast for at least 20 hours, as Brad Pilon suggests.

The reason why many aren't able to sustain it is that they go all gung ho when they start fasting intermittently—not thinking that fasting is a serious business. They get discouraged when they aren't able to sustain their fast long enough to complete it and drop it altogether. By starting with baby steps and gradually increasing those steps, you'll have a much higher shot at being able to sustain your IF protocol long enough to experience weight loss and other health benefits.

Hypoglycemia

Intermittent fasting results in lower blood sugar levels. But for diabetics, this may not be beneficial. They can't afford to go hungry for extended periods of time because, otherwise, their blood sugar levels may drop so low to the point of hypoglycemia. While low blood sugar is generally good, very low blood sugar levels—especially for diabetics—aren't.

So, you should ditch the idea of fasting intermittently if you have diabetes or are already prediabetic. Or if you really want to do the eat-stop-eat or other IF protocols, consult with your doctor first.

Other Possible Side Effects

Other minor side effects—especially at the beginning—may include:

- Acne

- Brain fog

- Caffeine addiction (which may lead to insomnia)

- Constipation

- Feeling bloated

- Headaches

- Heartburn

- Loose bowel movement

- Low energy

- Mood swings

- Stronger-than-usual hunger pangs

Reducing Potential Side Effects

Many of the potential side-effects can be easy to reduce or address. Some of the practical ways by which you can do so include:

For Constipation: You have to drink lots of water or calorie-free liquids and during your eating windows, eat foods with high dietary fiber content or supplement with psyllium fiber. If constipation persists, stop fasting and see your doctor.

For Bloating: You have to include soluble fiber in what you eat during your eating windows, or take a mild laxative to address bloating during your IF.

For Heartburn: Minimize the consumption of acid blockers and fatty food to stop heartburn, which normally happens at the beginning of an IF. If you feel the need to take acid blockers, check with your doctor about which you can eat and inform them that you're doing IF.

For Acne: Minimize consumption of high-fat and high-sugar foods on your eating days to minimize or stop acne.

Eating Frequently Is Better for Your Metabolism

It is nothing but a misconception that you need to keep frequently snacking to improve your metabolism. If you keep eating frequently, you will only be providing your body with a constant source of glucose and will prevent your body from burning any internal fat. Whenever you eat something, your body only uses a small portion of that food as energy and the rest is stored as fat for later use. When you keep eating, you are merely increasing the fat reserves in the body. So, you need to reduce your calorie intake and give your body a break if you want it to burn the energy stored within. Your body needs a little energy to digest and absorb the food you consume. About 10% of the calories you consume go toward this, and it is referred to as the thermic effect of food. So, if you consume 2,000 calories, the thermic effect of food is 200 calories. Regardless of whether you consume these calories at once or in 3 meals, the thermic effect stays the same. Therefore, it is safe to say that your body's metabolism doesn't slow down when you limit your calorie intake.

Causes Nutrient Deficiencies

There is a list of nutrients that your body needs. As long as you ensure that the food you consume has all the necessary nutrients, you don't have to worry about nutrient deficiencies. Consuming healthy and well-balanced meals while following the 5:2 diet protocol will ensure your body gets all the nutrients it needs. The trouble starts when you don't eat nutrient-dense foods and munch on unhealthy foods instead. You do need to adhere to the calorie restriction aspect of IF. However, it doesn't mean that you eat a packet of chips on a fasting day and then expect the diet to work. Doing this might lead to weight loss, but it will certainly deprive your body of the essential nutrients.

Loss of Muscle Mass

Protein catabolism occurs when there is a depletion of glycogen in the liver, which leads to loss of muscle mass. Simply put, at such a stage, your body will start to cannibalize its muscle tissue, and the amino acids present within are converted into glucose to support your body. When your body starts running out of these essential amino acids, it looks for other sources of them. If you deprive your body of glucose for over 28 hours, only then will your body start digesting its muscles. Up until then, you have nothing to worry about. While following the 5:2 diet, you will merely need to reduce your calorie intake, so you don't have to worry about losing muscle mass. In fact, by following this diet and combining it with the necessary exercises, you can build lean muscle.

Eating Disorders

If you stick to your diet and consume wholesome meals, you don't have to worry about developing any eating disorders. If you want to maintain a healthy relationship with food, then you must consume healthy meals without skimping on the necessary nutrients. However, if you ever suffered from an eating disorder in the past, are recovering from one, or are suffering from an eating disorder, then don't diet unless your doctor thinks it is safe for you to do so.

Causes Fertility Troubles for Women

Women tend to have different nutrient requirements than men. Some people tend to believe that intermittent fasting causes fertility issues for women. Well, this is nothing more than a misconception. Unless you are pregnant or lactating, then this diet is safe for a healthy adult woman to follow. While following this diet, you must ensure that you are carefully following the protocols mentioned and fast responsibly.

CHAPTER 12: HOW FASTING CHANGES THE MIND AND THE BODY

Regardless of whether one fasts for religious or health reasons, during the fasting period, changes in body and mind occur that could not really be explained in earlier times. They can now be scientifically proven. And the experts were also very fascinated by the processes they were able to measure in people who were fasting.

Auto Phagocytosis = Recycling of Waste Materials in the Cells

Auto phagocytosis or autophagy describes the self-digestion and recycling of cell components and waste materials that arise in the cells. This process is a natural process in the body, which generally works without fasting. It gets worse and worse as a person ages, which can promote the development of tumors. However, it was found that intermittent fasting can additionally support this cleansing process, regardless of age. After about 12 hours of fasting, the body increasingly resorts to the waste in order to convert it into new, first-class building material. Certain digestive enzymes are responsible for this.

This discovery, which brought the Japanese Auto phagocytosis the Nobel Prize in Medicine in 2016, could now conclusively explain why almost no muscle mass is lost during fasting.

Fat Loss through Ketones

The ketones are responsible for another biochemical miracle. These fatty acid molecules have a very central role when it comes to weight loss. This is because they arise when fat deposits are broken down and enable the human body to gain energy from these fats. In general, it is much easier for the body to use carbohydrates for energy production, which are normally also consumed in large quantities in the daily diet. But this is exactly where the problem lies. Because if you constantly supply the body with more than the required amounts of fuel, it simply doesn't seem to make sense to access fat reserves for energy.

In the meantime, it has been found that the breakdown of fat reserves begins after around 12 hours of fasting. The researchers were fascinated to find that the body evaluates the existing deposits differently and does not mine them evenly. Fat pads on the buttocks or the female breast are something like the iron reserve that is only tackled shortly before starvation. On the other hand, belly fat, which most people find visually annoying and is even classified as dangerous by doctors, is a comparatively easily accessible store. With some support, positive changes can even be noticed in a short time. These changes can be admired in the mirror, as they ensure a more beautiful figure, an improved body feeling, and more self-confidence. The internal processes are actually even more interesting. Because belly fat is partly responsible for cardiovascular diseases, type II diabetes, and inflammatory processes within the body. The coatings released by the belly fat, which are inflammatory messenger substances, are responsible for this. At the same time, the belly fat ensures the production of certain inhibitors that prevent the natural dissolution of blood clots. In the worst case, these can grow to a vascular-clogging size and lead to life-threatening embolisms or infarcts. Indirectly, belly fat is also attributed to a cancer-promoting effect, although this relationship has not yet been fully explored by science.

The relationship between belly fat and the natural feeling of satiety after eating is more clearly understood. Actually, the hormone leptin reports to the brain after a certain amount of food ingestion; it tells the brain, "Please don't eat anymore; I'm full." Excess belly fat suppresses the effect of this hormone, which is why fat people can often shovel in masses of calories. Of course, these are calories that are not needed in this amount and keep the vicious circle going.

While it has been proven that the keto diet helps in converting the existing body fat into the energy that the body really needs—how to deal with this finding is a moot point in the research community. There are some serious scientists who advocate the ketogenic diet. This means a serious change in diet, which in the ketogenic diet should mainly consist of fats and proteins, but hardly any carbohydrates.

We are also happy to point out that patients with certain symptoms (such as special forms of epilepsy) experience significant relief from the ketogenic diet—even if strong medications show little or no effect.

The community of critics is, however, much larger, and for good reasons. They point out that the purely ketogenic diet is merely an emergency program that was never intended for normal everyday use. The ketogenic diet, often called the "Stone Age diet," can even be downright dangerous in the long run. In particular, attention is drawn to the acidification of the body, which is massively boosted by the consumption of meat and animal fats. The kidneys barely manage to remove the excess of acids that are formed (they are therefore permanently exposed to the highest levels of stress), but some of the acids are still exhaled through the lungs. This, too, is actually an emergency program, but followers of a no-carb diet are generally noticeable in bad breath. Here the emergency has become the norm, which cannot go well in the long run.

However, this does not describe all of the risks and side effects of the keto diet. Since calcium is removed from the bones by chronic acidification, there is an increased risk of bone fractures and osteoporosis.

With intermittent fasting, the advantages of a ketogenic diet can be optimally used without having to accept the risks and side effects of a purely ketogenic diet described here.

Anti-Cancer Effect

Let's come back to the cancer-inhibiting effect of intermittent fasting. Here, among other things, it could be shown in animal experiments that the growth of cancer cells can be slowed down by intermittent fasting. Based on these findings, a study was carried out at the "Berlin Charité" with 34 women who had breast or ovarian cancer. Intermittent fasting showed not only a cancer-inhibiting effect but also a better tolerance to chemotherapy.

Scientifically sound findings on this phenomenon are still pending, but some explanations seem (to the experts) to go in the right direction. Healthy body cells seem to assume a kind of passive state during fasting, while cancer cells remain active and grow. In this way, they also make themselves vulnerable to the substances specifically used in chemotherapy, while the healthy cells have virtually taken cover. It has also been proven that cancer cells primarily need short-chain carbohydrates as a source of energy for their activity—these are mainly sugar and white flour products. The tumor cells, which are actually programmed to grow, find no or only very little sugar in the blood during the fasting periods, which means that the cells can be starved over time. However, serious science sees it as merely a supportive effect in cancer therapy, but not as an alternative to surgery, radiation, or chemotherapy.

Influence on Insulin Levels

A special focus in intermittent fasting is on insulin. Most people know "proteohormone" mainly from the fact that diabetics have to give it to themselves by external injections. This need arises from the fact that the human body needs insulin to digest carbohydrates. It is released from the pancreas as needed. Accordingly, diabetics have to make sure that they inject the right dose of insulin at the right moment in order to avoid dangerous hypoglycemia or hypoglycemia.

If the body gets used to switching to fat digestion, at least temporarily as in intermittent fasting, this relieves the pancreas. Increased insulin sensitivity will also develop over time. In other words, the amount of insulin needed to digest a certain amount of carbohydrates decreases with intermittent fasting.

The hormone glucagon is also of interest in this context. While insulin can help store large amounts of energy supplied through food in the form of body fats, the glucagon ensures that it is transported in the opposite direction. The glucagon is, therefore, largely responsible for the loss of fat during intermittent fasting—and this is a well-known effect of this type of diet.

Effect on the Intestinal Flora

The intestinal flora is particularly supported by intermittent fasting. Again, there are several aspects that work together in intermittent fasting. Above all, the resting state of the digestive organs allows the intestinal bacteria a recovery and regeneration phase. It can be observed here that healthy intestinal bacteria multiply rapidly, while the number of those that cause illness is kept to a minimum. This shows that the 16:8 rules (fasting 16 hours a day and eating 8 hours) are particularly good for the intestinal flora. However, this effect can also be determined with other rhythms of intermittent fasting.

Effect on the Brain

The brain also benefits from intermittent fasting because the human control center, in particular, depends on the type and intervals of food intake. "You are what you eat!" Naturally also refers to the appearance and physical well-being as a whole. But the brain is largely responsible for the characteristics that make up a person. This is due to hormones, the level of which is influenced by intermittent fasting. The positive effects on the course of Alzheimer's disease and other forms of dementia found in animal experiments with mice have not yet been conclusively explained. It is also unclear to what extent these observations can be transferred to humans. Nevertheless, it seems reasonable to assume that affected people can also benefit from intermittent fasting. It may even be possible to effectively prevent the diseases mentioned in this way.

These effects are primarily attributed to the protein BDNF ("brain-derived neurotrophic factor"), which is released after a period of at least 12 hours of fasting. This protein forms a natural protection for the nerve cells.

Furthermore, the ketones produced by intermittent fasting must be mentioned again, which are the brain's absolute favorite food. Even glucose, which is said to be a real energy booster, especially in the form of grape sugar, is only the second choice after ketones. It has been shown that these ketones also have a positive effect on the nerve connections in the brain, particularly the hippocampus. The ketones ensure that people learn better and can remember many things more easily.

Antiaging

Intermittent fasting is antiaging from the inside out. The Italian-American gerontologist Valtier Longo made amazing discoveries in the blood of fasters. During the fasting period, the number of white blood cells decreases, which is due to the recycling of old immune cells. At the same time, new cells are formed, which clearly supports the immune system. This renewal mechanism is actually already in the cradle and works even without fasting. However, it weakens as age increases, which is why older people are usually more susceptible to diseases. Regular fasting does not completely stop the aging process that can be seen here; however, it is slowed down significantly. The lowering of an enzyme called protein kinase A (PKA)—identified by Valtier Longo's team—is also helpful. This makes it easier for the body to activate the self-renewal of the stem cells. All of this leads to improved health and an extended lifespan.

And it should actually be clear to everyone that the application of certain creams can cosmetically change the appearance, and in some cases, a medical effect on the skin can also be demonstrated. But the skin is of course not the only organ that is subject to the aging process. It is better to stimulate the entire organism to renew itself.

CHAPTER 13: STARTING YOUR JOURNEY

By now, you know you need some balance in your life, but maybe you aren't sure how to start. To give a better idea, we are going to do a small exercise. Stand up and lift one of your feet off the floor. If you have a low balance, be sure to stand next to a wall just if you need a helping hand. When you feel like you're about to fall over, first try a quick, healthy physical correction to try to stay balanced. It might look like leaning to the opposite side drastically in an attempt to bring yourself back to the center. Woah! If you just tried this, you just experienced the adverse side effects of finding balance too aggressively. You probably fell off balance again, only in the opposite direction! Now, try again, and this time when you feel off-balance, slowly adjust only one part of your body at a time. Maybe this looks like pressing your foot on the ground is a little more challenging in the center. Maybe place one palm gently on the wall. You get the idea, finding and retaining balance works by adding and maintaining healthy lifestyle choices one step at a time.

Everything we have covered in this book works the same. If you are trying to eat healthier, start by making a list of your unhealthy eating habits. Every 2 weeks, remove one unhealthy food from your everyday diet. It will take patience, especially when starting a new health-improving journey. Most of us tend to get excited we changing and want to clean out our entire pantry and fridge. Remember, this is no different from aggressively leaning to one side in an attempt to find balance. The results will also be the same:

To crash! And you won't be able to retain the healthy lifestyle you're currently dreaming of. Always remember, one step at a time.

Finding Your Balance

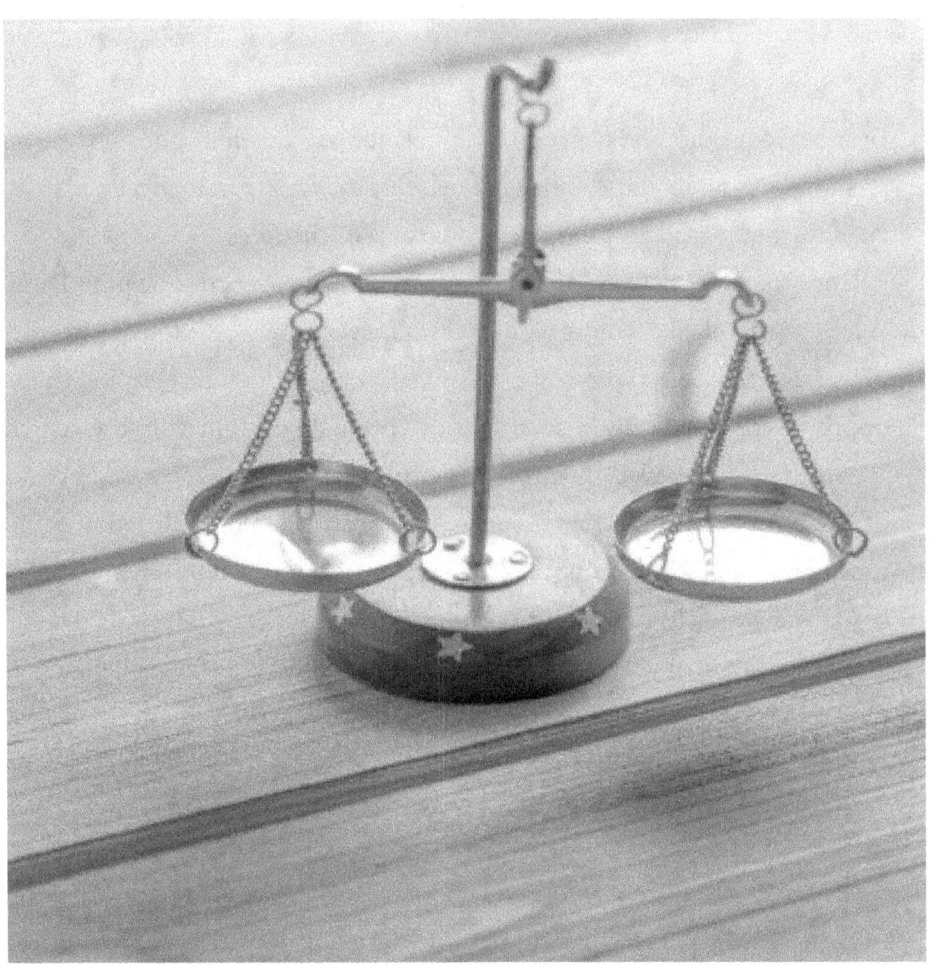

Step 1

Choose a fasting style that fits your everyday life. Remember, if you're used to eating from 9 a.m. to 10 p.m., it wouldn't be wise to choose a drastic fasting style. Some better options might be the 5:2, where you usually eat for 5 days out of the week and then limit yourself to only 500–700 calories on 2 nonconsecutive days. Another great fasting style is to try "time restricting" if this sounds like your current eating habits. In the morning, don't eat anything until you have had at least 3 glasses of water, your morning tea, or coffee, and wait until your stomach grumbles to be fed. You might be surprised by the time when your body feels like it needs food. Many people find that they don't actually feel hungry until 10 a.m., 11 a.m., or even noon! Once you find the time you feel hungry, go ahead and eat! Look at the clock and close your eating window after 8 or 10 hours. Below are some time examples for you to refer to:

- 10 a.m. to 8 p.m. (14-hour fast) or 10 a.m. to 6 p.m. (16-hour fast)

- 11 a.m. to 9 p.m. (14-hour fast) or 11 a.m. to 7 p.m. (16-hour fast)

- Noon to 10 p.m. (14-hour fast) or noon to 8 p.m. (16-hour fast)

Another reminder is that if you have a certain time for lunch at work, make sure to plan your fast around those hours. You need food for energy while you are at work, so you don't feel lethargic all day. You can also make your fast last longer or shorter, depending on your daily life schedule. Feel like 16 hours is too long? Adjust it to 14. Do you feel like 16 hours isn't enough? Try 18.

For the 5:2 fasting style, remember to choose your fasting days as the least active days in your week. Start noticing what days of the week are slower-paced, more relaxed, and choose those as the days where you limit your calories. If you choose a more active day to reduce your calories, you may risk some adverse side effects of fasting, such as lightheadedness, lack of energy, trouble focusing, and intense food cravings.

If your lifestyle calls for a more advanced fasting method, or if you eat a lot and find yourself grazing rather than eating big meals, you may want to choose alternate day fasting. That doesn't mean that you can't eat anything on the days you are fasting, just like the 5:2 style; merely limiting your calorie intake on those days works as well. Being a grazer would work well with this style because your fast won't feel that different from your regular days. You will just need to be more calorie-conscious of what you're grazing on.

Step 2

Listen to how your body reacts to certain foods to create your perfect nutrition style. If you don't know where to start with this, start testing your digestive system on the following foods: Dairy, wheat, gluten, meat, spice, and seafood. For a week, try each of these categories separately to ensure you know what specific food is causing your body harm or harmony!

Also, don't forget to drink the dang water! No matter if you're eating foods that work well with your body, if you aren't drinking enough water, you're going to feel bloated, constipated, and tired. Water is your new magic potion to wellness!

Step 3

Don't forget to add your favorite type of activity a few times a week to keep your body's wellness balanced! Depending on your lifestyle and where you are in your life, you'll want to focus more on cardio or resistance training activities. You can always vary your workouts to ensure you don't get bored or feel like you have to 'work out.' The goal is to view these activities as something fun you look forward to, and that will release some awesome endorphins for your day!

Step 4

Listen to your body and how it's reacting to your new lifestyle. If you choose a fasting style, activity, or foods that may not be right for you, your body will let you know! Start writing down how you feel during the day until you find the perfect balance. If you don't do this, odds are you won't get it right the first time, and it won't last.

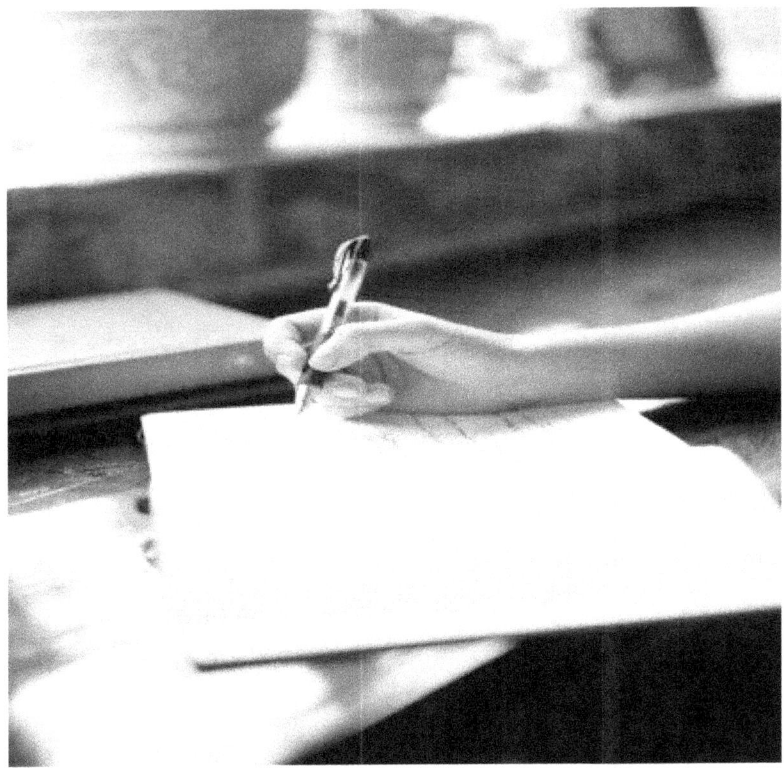

CHAPTER 14: INTERMITTENT FASTING VERSUS OTHER DIETS

As mentioned earlier, even if intermittent fasting can help you lose weight, it is not a diet in itself. It is a fasting method and is accompanied by a diet, and the diet should be a healthy one.

Intermittent Fasting versus Calorie Counting

This is a close comparison because it is important to pay attention to calorie intake even if you fast intermittently. The difference between intermittent fasting and calorie counting is that no matter which type of intermittent fasting method you choose, fasting is the main driver of this strategy.

When using the 5:2 method, men and women are encouraged to limit their calorie intake to 600 and 500 calories, respectively. This fact is with every meal after the fast. Even within the fasting regime, it would be inevitable that the calorie intake will be reduced.

However, there is no doubt that calorie counting is a successful diet, but it means a bit more work than when you chose intermittent fasting. With the latter, you will automatically reduce calories, while with a calorie-counting diet, you must measure and calculate your daily intake

Intermittent Fasting versus Intermittent Energy Restriction (IER) Strategies

The difference is that intermittent fasting is the restriction of food for a period of time. This is followed by an extended period within which you would eat; for example, within a 4-hour window.

In contrast with intermittent fasting, intermittent energy restriction strategies restrict energy intake to a window of 8–10 hours each day. One big difference is that this is a static way of 'fasting' compared to the different ways of intermittent fasting.

This also means that you have more leeway in intermittent fasting, as intermittent energy restriction strategies will limit your daily consumption to as much as 25% of your energy needs. "With intermittent fasting, you can limit your energy intake by 60–100% on the day of the fast and eat as much as possible when the fast is over." (Renders, Corey A et al 2019).

Intermittent Fasting versus the Keto Diet

The keto diet, which is short for the ketogenic diet, has become as popular as intermittent fasting. The keto diet involves control over your carbohydrates. For some people, this means that your daily carbohydrate (carbs) intake should be less than 50 grams. Others go as low as between 10–20 grams. As with any diet, if you restrict your nutritional intake, and if you choose the keto diet, then you need to consult a doctor.

With intermittent fasting, you restrict yourself to "eating windows." You have a choice of what you eat within these windows, and can then choose to restrict your carbs or your calories during this time. However, with keto, you restrict your carbs to less than 50 grams each day, which can lead to nutritional deficiencies.

"Intermittent fasting gives you more freedom to decide what food to eat, but the keto diet may restrict your diet, and social and psychological difficulties for some people." (Munns 2019).

In recent years, the keto diet has become more mainstream than most of the surrounding diets. It has developed to the point of having specific products ascribed to the diet, and some of the products are quite prescriptive as well. As said earlier, intermittent fasting gives you more freedom of choices to choose your foods according to your lifestyle as well.

Intermittent Fasting versus Traditional Diets

At this point, you already have a sufficient understanding of what intermittent fasting is all about. Even though we are pitting it against traditional diets, this are exactly the diets you might want to include in your eating window.

Examples of traditional diets you might want to include in your intermittent fasting regime are:

The Mediterranean Diet

The Mediterranean diet is called this as it covers the traditional foods and means of the people around the Mediterranean Sea. Some of the foods include fruits, vegetables, whole grains, nuts, beans, herbs, spices, and healthy fats. Olive oil is one of the good fats for this diet. It is important to include fish and seafood in this diet at least twice a week. Other foods include fermented dairies, such as yogurt and traditional cheese (like feta), eggs, and poultry. Red meat and sweets are rarely eaten, and water and wine play a key role.

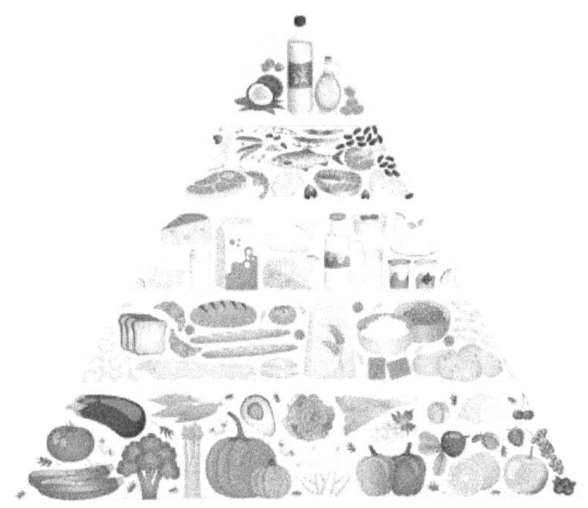

Mediterranean Food Pyramid (Free Image from Apixaban)

The African Heritage Diet

The African heritage diet is based on the healthy eating habits of African countries. In addition to being nutritious, these foods are traditionally delicious. Therefore, a meal based on African traditions will be a feast for you. Some of these deliciously healthy foods have their roots in Jamaica and Nigeria. In the US, the French-Creole foods are fusions of delicious African heritage diets.

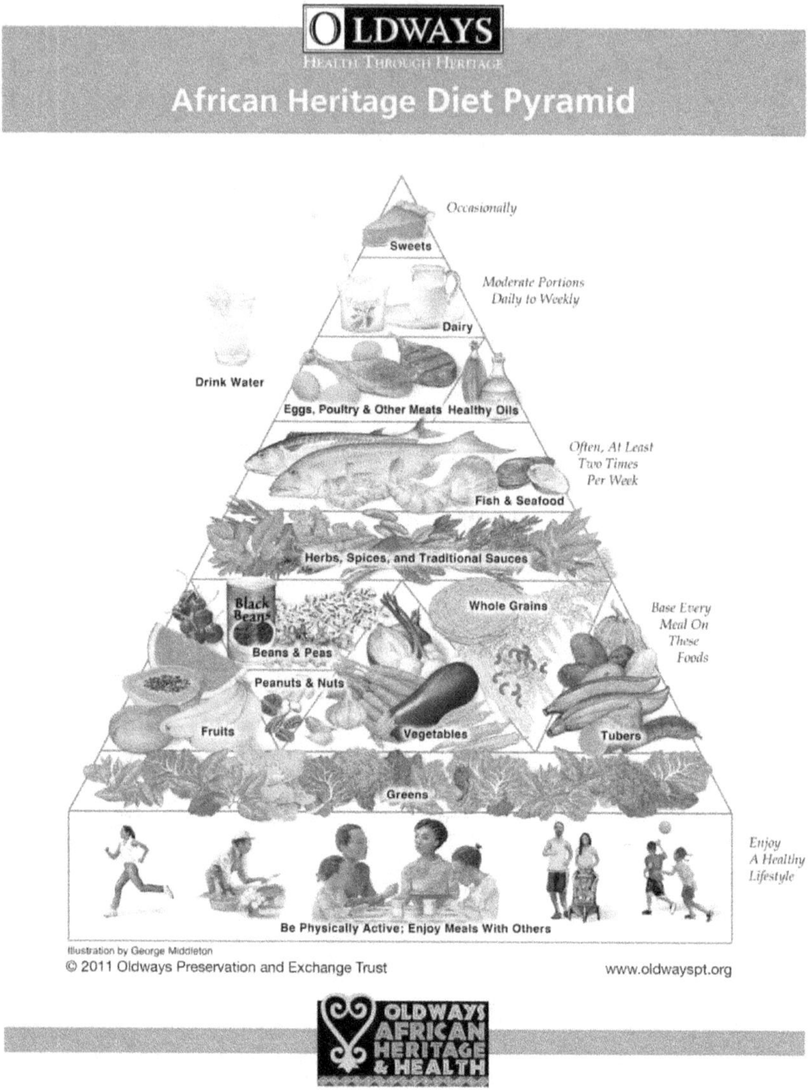

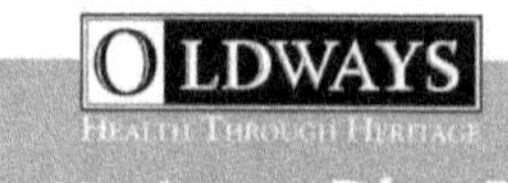

African Heritage Diet Pyramid

Latin American Heritage Diet

This diet is based on South American traditions, including Portuguese, Spanish, and large-scale variations of the indigenous peoples of the Mayans, Aztecs, Incas, and many other surrounding countries (called Latin America). The cultures contributed to a pyramid that offers nutrition but also delicious cuisine.

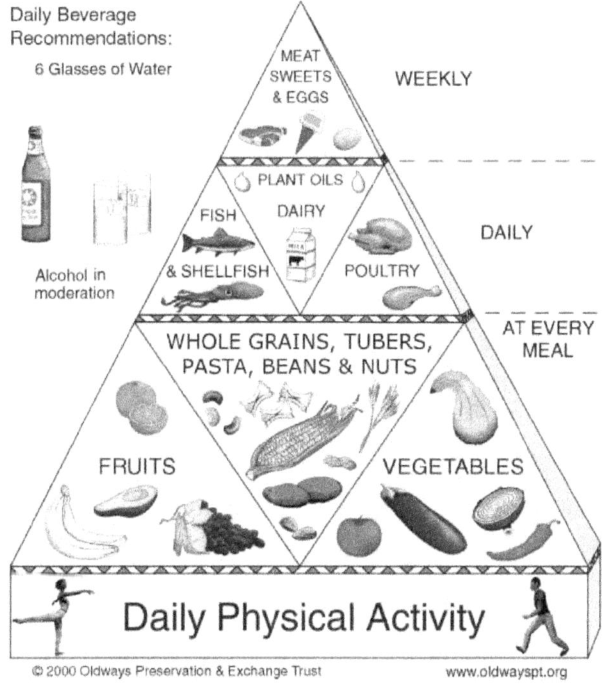

Latin American Food Pyramid

The delicious foods mentioned in the pyramids above should serve as motivation for the eating window of your intermittent fasting. However, it should also not distract you from your goals.

CHAPTER 15: MASTERING YOUR EMOTIONS TO PREVENT THEM FROM MASTERING YOU

Now we have an opportunity to get our thinking straight. Whether it's in world history or in an individual, every great leap forward begins with a single idea. Here, our focus is on better health and losing weight. When we start fasting, we will have an effective strategy to accomplish something that has eluded us in the past. Beyond that, we must be sure that our actions are broadly in line with our values and responsibilities. If they are not, things will go haywire again, either with our food or in some other area of our lives. Haven't we always known that it wasn't just about food?

There is a trio of tools that are essential for this work. They are "focus," "routine," and "self-discipline." No, not the white-knuckle willpower that we employed in the past when we were dieting, which never worked for long and is just another word for self-bullying. "Self-discipline," on the other hand, is a gentler creature that never tries to beat us into submission, but instead, takes our concerns on board and reasons with us like a wise parent. "Routine," also mild-mannered, is what allows us to get up each morning without having to face the task of 'reinventing the wheel' for that particular day. Certain features of our lives can be fixed in a pattern that suits us when we have routine and discipline. We don't have to think much about them as long as they continue to serve us and don't unduly upset those around us. "Focus" is what gives our lives meaning and is the reason we employ the other tools. Together these tools reduce our everyday stresses to a minimum.

Self-discipline provides structure in our lives and gives us the ability to make the best choices for ourselves at any given moment. It brings stability and calm, keeping us moving toward the goals that we've set for ourselves. When we start fasting, we will see that it calls for commitment. Self-discipline, focus, and routine lead us to commitment and ultimately to success in almost anything we set out to achieve. It may be a person, such as a spouse or a personal assistant who takes care of things, but it can also be a sensible daily routine around which their lives run smoothly.

In some respects, our lives may have become chaotic, but through self-discipline and routine, we can set ourselves up with an environment of calm that gives us the chance to rediscover "peace of mind." In this kind of 'headspace,' we can find reserves of energy and courage that we never even knew we had. We can wake up each morning having a framework for the day ahead. It makes life far more manageable.

Your deep-seated beliefs and truths have been forming in your mind over the whole of your life. Thoughts, emotions, and lived experiences have made either positive or negative impressions on your psyche. They have created neural pathways within your brain, where nothing is ever really forgot. When our thoughts are positive, these beliefs and attitudes can serve us well, providing stability and keeping us grounded. At other times, however, our views and expectations can be crippling, holding us back or waiting to trip us up. The good news is, quite simply, that these beliefs are within our control. They are part of a fixed mindset that can be changed. The brain is an incredibly flexible instrument that can rebuild positive attitudes over time.

You may have heard of the "marshmallow test," which was performed on young children at "Stanford University" in the 1970s. It focused on the implications of delayed gratification versus instant gratification in the formulation of life skills. Essentially, children were told that they could have one marshmallow immediately or be rewarded with a second marshmallow later if they waited. Following the children in a longitudinal study, researchers found that the children who managed to wait for the reward were far more likely to be successful in various aspects of life. Crucially, for our purposes, they did much better at maintaining a healthy weight. Instant gratification leads to a quick, pleasurable dopamine rush to the brain, followed by an almost immediate crash. Self-discipline, on the other hand, can lead to meeting long-term goals that foster a more meaningful sense of happiness and purpose. Consider this in the context of weight loss. A year on, we probably won't remember the pizza and doughnuts we consumed one Saturday evening, despite the fleeting pleasure at the time. What we won't forget, and what will give us the most satisfaction and confidence is the success of our goal. And for us, that goal is lasting weight loss.

Exercising through Smart Goals

One of the main ways we can exercise the power of our minds is in building and maintaining better habits. Establishing goals is the best way I know to direct our efforts. They may sometimes feel like another burden on top of everything else, but having goals in place will eliminate stress. Not just any old goals, of course, but SMART goals that set out essential signposts at the start of our journey. SMART stand for "Specific," "Measurable," "Achievable," "Relevant," and "Timed." These are avenues to success that inspire and motivate us to achieve our goals. Lots of people, organizations, and businesses use them as a tried and tested method of accomplishing better results.

Specific

Turn your health and weight loss plans into specific goals through the following questions. Please do this exercise in your journal and supply your own answers.

- **Sample Question 1:** What do I hope to achieve?
- **Sample Answer 1:** I want to achieve effective and lasting weight loss in the context of a more fulfilled life.
- **Sample Question 2:** Why is this important to me?
- **Sample Answer 2:** Because, ultimately, I will be physically and psychologically healthier, have greater self-esteem, and more energy.
- **Sample Question 3:** What external resources do I need to succeed at this goal?
- **Sample answer 3:** I need Information and a supportive group of friends.
- **Sample Question 4:** What internal resources do I need?
- **Sample Answer 4:** I need to develop my mental strength and determination, ditch self-pity, and try to be more optimistic. If others can do it, then so can I.
- **Sample Question 5:** What limitations do I face, and how do I overcome them?
- **Sample Answer 5:** Think of your limits as minor obstacles.

Join our Facebook group, read this book, and find other online resources. When we ask the universe for what we want, it will be supplied.

Measurable

You know that losing weight takes time. You will lose weight when you start intermittent fasting, but be patient and make a record of the date you started fasting and your starting weight.

Achievable

The "S" in "SMART" also stands for 'Small' because a series of small goals is best. What it doesn't stand for is 'sabotage!' I can say that setting unachievable or unrealistic goals is just a sure way to fail. Be kind to yourself and grant yourself the time and space to make these positive changes, especially in light of your other duties and responsibilities. We are all works in progress!

Relevant

Your goals must take the other people in your life into account. Stay in alignment with your fundamental values, current situation, and your relationships. It must also take your needs into account. Self-love is a core value, don't forget. Use your journal to get your priorities sorted out.

Timed

Any achievable goal must have a deadline—but be flexible and kind to yourself. Distinguish between short, medium, and long-term goals and don't limit yourself to just weight loss. After all, that's only one part of your life. As before, use your journal to track your progress.

116

I ask that you will do your part by being as honest with yourself as you can. Being open to new ideas, and sometimes ready to suspend your disbelief, will ensure that you get the maximum benefit from this book.

Ask yourself if the time has now come to finally relinquish the past. Anger, frustration and fury, and blaming others, our parents, our partners, or our work colleagues, are all a terrible waste of time. Worse, they hold us back from getting on with our potentially great lives. Sorting ourselves out by using our available headspace to be inspired by our potential future and to help others is a much better idea. To achieve greatness, we need mind strength and character strength. Self-pity is the antithesis of these good qualities. I believe that it is the one quality that holds most people back from their destiny. Drop it now if you can. This is the time to make a real and lasting change.

Continue using your journal to measure your progress. Writing is one of the most effective ways to examine your feelings, thoughts, and habits. Mae West famously claimed that we should all "keep a diary because someday it'll keep you."

Start writing your weight story in your journal. When did you start to feel that your weight was a problem? Write about how and when you got fat, and explain that you no longer need your weight because you now have better ways of protecting yourself than you did before. At last, you have more control over your life. Write in detail about all of the disadvantages of being fat, now and in the past. How did it affect your relationships with your significant others, your children, and your mother? Did it have negative consequences for your health? Did it hold you back in your job or career?

Your journal is a work in progress, just as you are. Keep your journal handy, and try to write something in it at least a few times a week. Let it turn into a record of your growth for you to become the person you want to be. Set up your weight loss goals, using the SMART goal guidelines.

Food for Thought

Many years ago, one of my teachers, a nun called sister Immaculata, used to tell us that, "Our emotions are great servants but terrible masters." To take the actions we need to take, we sometimes need to put our emotions on ice and think things through in a cool, logical way. As with other skills, practice makes, if not perfect, then acceptable—which is better than perfect.

Thinking things through is a much sounder basis for action than going by our feelings alone. Our emotions can be volatile and changeable like the weather. "Thinking things through carefully" means that we are far less likely to make mistakes.

Through mindfulness, we can harness the strength of our thoughts and take control of our emotions and actions. Cultivating discipline is a significant part of progress toward lasting weight loss. We can make a pact with time by turning away from instant gratification in the expectation of more satisfying, long-term success. Forging new habits and routines becomes exciting as we build up our psychological muscles. Building and maintaining better and healthier habits using SMART goals gives us a road map for our journey.

CHAPTER 16: INTERMITTENT FASTING FAQS

Taking note of your caloric intake and removing carbohydrates from your meals are all forms of diet. However, the kind of diet that is currently in vogue does not limit the kind of food you eat; instead, it is focused on the time of day in which you eat.

This kind of diet is known as intermittent fasting, and for some time now, it has gone up so much that it is recognized as a popular dietary technique amongst other forms of diet. At the moment, intermittent fasting has become one of the most sought-after kinds of diet.

One may be curious as to why intermittent fasting has become so well known. The reason is that "It seems a lot easier for some people," as Dr. Elizabeth Lowden, MD put it, a bariatric endocrinologist at the Northwestern Medicine Metabolic Health and Surgical Weight Loss Center at Delnor Hospital in Geneva, Illinois.

Below are some of the asked questions on intermittent fasting and the answers to them.

What Is Intermittent Fasting and How Is It Different from Starvation?

Intermittent fasting is a way to eat in which you take turns between eating at a certain time and fasting—or reducing substantially the number of calories that you take in. The difference between other kinds of diet and intermittent fasting is that with other kinds of diet, you eat specific foods.

What's more important is that intermittent fasting does not mean that you have to keep yourself from eating. Intermittent fasting, instead, means that you eat your repast (meals) at a specific time, and then for the remaining part of the day, whereas you will fast in the night.

What Is the History of Intermittent Fasting?

In August 2015, a published study in the "**Journal of the Academy of Nutrition and Dietetics**" showed that fasting had been a practice since antediluvian times and most people who practiced fasting were religious people.

What made intermittent fasting widely known was a documentary broadcasted in the year 2012 titled "**Eat, Fast and Live Longer.**" It was also around the same time period that many books on intermittent fasting were printed and published according to the "**Journal of the Academy of Nutrition and Dietetics,**" and one of the books that brought about the popularity of the concept was "**The Fast Diet,**" published in 2013.

Sara Gottfried, the author of "**Brain-Body Diet**," based in Berkeley, California, stated that "Over the past five years, rigorous research has shown the remarkable benefits of intermittent fasting, which is behind this sudden interest."

How Does Intermittent Fasting Work?

According to "Harvard Health," the basic idea of intermittent fasting is that you set a particular time period every week in which you eat, and a certain period of time when you would neither eat nor drink (or what you eat and drink would be limited to a great extent) in spite of the type or version of intermittent fasting you are following.

Different Types of Intermittent Fasting?

There are various versions (types) of intermittent fasting, and in all of them, the day or the week is split into time periods where food is eaten and when fasting is practiced. During the period of fasting, you could not eat at all, or you can eat only a small quantity of food. The most common intermittent fasting versions include:

The 16:2 Version: People who follow this version of intermittent fasting don't eat breakfast and restrict the period of time in which they eat to 8 hours a day, and fast for the remaining 16 hours. They either decide to eat between 11 a.m. and 7 p.m. or between 12 p.m. and 8 p.m.—or even between 1 p.m. and 9 p.m. This version is also referred to as the "lean gains protocol."

Alternate-Day Fasting: According to a published study in October 2014 in Translational Research, this version of intermittent fasting requires that the number of calories that is usually consumed be reduced by 25%, then the following day the normal way of eating should be followed. It means, on day one, you eat normally, and the next day, you reduce calorie intake by 25%, then the next day, you eat normally, and then on and on.

Eat-Fast-Eat: In this version of intermittent fasting, 24 hours is used for fasting in a week; it could be once or twice depending on the individual and the results they intend to get. Basically, in this version, you don't eat dinner or any meal for one day until it is dinner time the following day.

The 5:2 Version: In this version of intermittent fasting, 2 nonconsecutive days are chosen as the days of fasting in which only about 400—600 calories should be consumed. On the remaining 5 days of that week, there are no eating restrictions.

All the above versions of intermittent fasting will help you lose some pounds when you consistently follow the diet and bring to a minimum the number of calories you consume.

The 16:2 version is the major type or version of intermittent fasting that is practiced worldwide because many believe it to be easier to follow this diet than all the other diets. It is also very simple and bearable.

Can Intermittent Fasting Help You Lose Weight?

Weight loss is possible when one begins to practice intermittent fasting in the sense that it forces you to not eat between meals and also reduce the intake of calories, and when you do that, your body has no choice but to rely on the fat it had stored in the cells to get energy.

As this happens, the hormone levels in the body will change; for example, the release of norepinephrine (noradrenaline), which is the hormone that burns fat, will be increased, and insulin will be reduced, thus allowing for the increase in the level of hormones that facilitate growth.

As a result of the changes in the hormone levels in the body, fasting for a short time will increase the rate of metabolism in the body by about 3.6–14 or 15%. The way by which intermittent fasting causes one to lose weight is by changing the equation of calorie intake—it does this by forcing you to consume fewer calories and burn more.

All that intermittent fasting boils down to is the restriction in the intake of calories. Basically, when people only have a limited amount of time to eat a day, they will undoubtedly consume a lesser quantity of calories on that day than when they are allowed to eat—in the way and manner they please for the whole day.

All the types of intermittent fasting prevent the consumption of meals after a certain amount of time, like 7 p.m. This also has an added advantage in that it prevents people from eating at night, which has been shown by various studies to help with metabolic syndrome, obesity, and the development of belly fat—an example of such studies is the study that was published in December 2018 in **BMC Public Health.**"

The same study of 2014 showed that people who engaged in intermittent fasting lost about 4—7% of the circumference of their waists, which indicates that harmful belly fat—which works up to around the organs and brings about diseases—was lost.

Another study that was conducted revealed that through intermittent fasting, less muscle was lost in comparison to the general method of totally restricting a certain amount of calorie consumption.

Do not forget that the major reason that intermittent fasting is successful when it comes to weight loss is that you only get to eat a smaller quantity of calories in general. If you decide to consume a great number of calories during the periods when you are allowed to eat, you may never get to lose any weight.

There is some opinion that the amount of weight people lose when they practice intermittent fasting is not substantially different from the result obtained following diets that totally restrict a specific percentage of calories. A study that was published in November 2018 in the "American Journal of Clinical Nutrition" discovered that a diet that cut the consumption of calories by 20% produced the same result in terms of weight loss as the 5:2 version of intermittent fasting in a year. All the same, the method of intermittent fasting for weight loss is easier to follow than other dieting techniques.

What Are the Benefits of Intermittent Fasting and Are They Legit?

Below are some of the benefits to be anticipated when engaging in intermittent fasting.

A study published in 2018 in "Nutrition and Healthy Aging" noted the possibility that alternate-day fasting may lead to a greater result in regard to weight loss than that of eating under time restrictions, although it would be harder to stick with alternate-day fasting than it would be with time-restricted eating.

Lengthens Life

A study, which was carried out involving animals and published in December 2014 in **"Cell,"** showed that a reduction in calorie intake has the potency of slowing down aging. Although the study has not been carried out on humans, there is a possibility the same results could be obtained.

Better Heart Health

The results of a study, which was published in "Nutrition Journal," showed that intermittent fasting helped the participants of the study to lose weight, lose fat, and also lower the levels of cholesterol in their bodies, and because of these, the researchers who conducted the study came to the conclusion that engaging in intermittent fasting can help reduce the risk of suffering from coronary artery disease.

Reduces Insulin Resistance

A study, which was published in February 2014 in **"Frontiers of Medicine,"** revealed that insulin resistance is the trademark of type II diabetes and obesity—being corpulent—can bring about a rise in insulin resistance.

On the other hand, a study published in **Nutrients** in April 2019 showed that intermittent fasting could reduce insulin resistance by bringing about a reduction in the number of calories a person consumes.

CONCLUSION

Intermittent fasting is a beautiful way to lose weight without cutting calories. Not only does it help you lose weight, but it enables you to keep it off, too. Intermittent fasting is useful because your body doesn't have time to get used to eating less. That means that you're going to lose weight every time you fast for some time.

While intermittent fasting is a low-calorie diet, you shouldn't view it as a diet. It's not a permanent solution—it's just an effective way to lose weight and maintain it, too. You can get intermittent fast any time of the day and still be successful.

Intermittent fasting will prevent your body from getting used to eating less by allowing you to eat normally during those 24-hour periods where you're not eating. When your body doesn't have time to adjust, it doesn't get used to eating fewer calories.

Whether you choose 4 hours or 8 hours, no matter how long your fast lasts, you're going to lose weight. One study found that participants who did 4-hour fasts lost 25% more weight in 2 weeks than those who did 8-hour fasts!

Intermittent fasting is a diet strategy that allows you to activate autophagy, an essential cellular process in which longer-lived cells or organelles are removed for recycling.

This study shows that intermittent fasting (or intermittent calorie restriction) is a way to extend lifespan in animals and humans. It allows you to eat less while you still get your daily calorie requirement. This eating schedule will help you lose weight and boost your metabolism.

Intermittent fasting is beneficial for those who are insulin-resistant or have diabetes. It will increase your insulin sensitivity, which can help you keep your blood sugar level under control. Also, it can help you reduce your risk of developing diabetes by up to 80%.

Intermittent fasting benefits are the subject of great debate. While there is some anecdotal evidence, scientific research has yet to uncover definitive answers. However, there is enough evidence to show that intermittent fasting can provide some benefits.

First, intermittent fasting can be a very healthy habit for people who consume more calories than they burn. Additionally, it can produce ketosis—a state in which the body uses fat as its primary energy source instead of glucose. It's also been shown to induce adaptations in the brain as well as other organs. While these adaptations have been observed in mice and rats, they don't provide concrete information about how intermittent fasting affects humans.